DANGEROUS TO YOUR HEALTH

Capitalism in Health Care

VICENTE NAVARRO

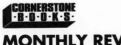

**MONTHLY REVIEW PRESS
NEW YORK**

Library of Congress Cataloging-in-Publication Data
Navarro, Vicente.
   Dangerous to your health : capitalism in health care / Vicente Navarro.
      p.   cm.
   Includes bibliographical references and index.
   ISBN 0-85345-864-2 : $22.00. — ISBN 0-85345-865-0 (pbk.) : $10.00
   1. Social medicine—United States. 2. Medical policy—United States. 3. Right to
health care—United States. 4. Medical care—United States. I. Title.
RA418.3.U6N38   1993
362.1'0973—dc20   93-21413
                                                          CIP

Monthly Review Press
122 West 27th Street
New York, NY 10001

Manufactured in the United States of America
10 9 8 7 6 5 4 3 2 1

To my father and my mother, who taught me,
through the example of their own lives, the
meaning of solidarity and freedom and the
struggle that is required to achieve both.

CONTENTS

INTRODUCTION

John Dunlop worked in the Bethlehem Steel mills in East Baltimore for over twenty years. Three years ago he was laid off, one of the 2,312 workers laid off from the mills in the last ten years. He not only lost his job: he also lost health insurance for himself and his family. He could no longer receive the care he needed for a heart condition because he could not afford the insurance. He died in May 1993 from a stroke. He was one of the 100,000 people who die in the United States each year because they cannot afford medical care.

Mary McCormick was an administrator at Maryland National Bank. Until about a year ago she thought her health insurance covered all the necessary medical and hospital care for herself and her family. She found out she was wrong. On January 27, 1992, she had a stroke that left her so seriously handicapped that she needed long-term care. But her health insurance did not include this benefit. She had to sell almost everything she owned to make herself eligible for government assistance. And in order to protect her husband's assets—their home and car—she had to divorce him. In March 1993 Mary killed herself. She was one of the 202 million people in the United States whose health benefits do not include long-term care. Many of these people assume they have such comprehensive coverage, only to find that this is not the case.

Anne Lorraine is one of the 120 people who wash the floors and make the beds at the Johns Hopkins Hospital and another hospital in Baltimore. She is an African-American who came to Baltimore from Charlottesville, South Carolina, twenty years ago, when she was ten years old. She lives with her mother and three children. But although she has two jobs, neither employer pays health benefits for her or her family and she cannot afford to pay the premiums herself. Thirty-two percent of all health care workers in the United States do not have health insurance. They are part of the 38 million Americans who face the same plight.

John Dunlop, Mary McCormick, and Anne Lorraine are representative of the millions of victims of the U.S. health care system. In no other developed country do people face such a cruel situation. Meanwhile, the powerful establishment and its hired pens proclaim that we have the "best system of medical care in the world." Health care is the largest industry in the United States. The components of the "medical-industrial complex"—the insurance companies, drug companies, hospital equipment companies, and the medical professions, among others—are among the most profitable companies in the country. The head of Mary McCormick's insurance company makes $2.5 million a year, and the director of one of the hospitals where Anne Lorraine works makes $800,000 a year. A lot of money is made in the house of medicine. In no other sector of our society is the wealth of the few so clearly based on the suffering of the many.

Why do we face such a situation? This book attempts to answer this enormously important question. The problems in the funding and delivery of health services are much in the news these days. Day after day the press covers the human drama caused by the failures of our health care system. Those in government and in the medical establishment are aware that people are angry and want change. We have seen the publication of hundreds of articles and books that try to show why medical care is so expensive and/or why so many people have problems getting insurance. Many of these are full of helpful information. But most focus on how different interest groups in medicine—the American Medical Association, the hospital industry, and others—operate. They do not address the root of the problem, which lies in the nature of our economic and social system.

In other words, we cannot understand the problems of our health care system by looking only at the actors and agents of its delivery. We need to understand that, contrary to official rhetoric, the moving force in health care delivery is not responding to people's needs but satisfying the greed of those who control the key institutions of our society, including health care. The economic and political order—capitalism—governs the financing and delivery of our health services. Indeed, it is business "entrepreneurship" that is the moving force behind our medical institutions. Here lies the root of the human tragedy behind the death and suffering of John Dunlop and Mary McCormick, and the precarious situation faced by Anne Lorraine and her family—and millions like them.

Why does this oppressive system continue? In a capitalist system, people are divided not only by race, gender, national origin, and religion but also by *class*. This point needs to be stressed because the United States is often portrayed as having no classes because the majority is middle class. Terms such as capitalist class, working class, and class struggle are dismissed as foreign. Vincent Canby, the senior film critic for the *New York Times,* recently concluded that a British film that details the lives of working-class men and women was irrelevant for U.S. audiences because "the United States does not have a working class."[1]

This view of the United States as a middle-class society is

profoundly ideological. But it confuses rather than clarifies our reality. As I will show in this book, not only does the United States have classes, but class is the most important category for explaining what happens in U.S. society and its health care system. Needless to say, other power categories, such as race and gender, have enormous importance as well. But in the current literature, including the progressive literature, class has been relegated to a secondary level. This book aims at restoring the key importance of class in explaining U.S. society and its medicine.

The book therefore begins with an examination of the patterns of class control of health care. It shows how the capitalist class (and its different components) has an enormous influence on the way in which health care is financed and delivered. The insurance companies and the large corporate employers are the major forces that shape this financing. Their economic and political influence is enormous, limiting considerably the government's ability to respond to popular demands. The lack of universal coverage, insufficient coverage, the relationship between coverage and employment, and many of the other problems of our health care system are rooted in the power of the corporate class.

Chapter 2 shows how the deterioration in health care, including the increase in the number of Americans who either have insufficient insurance or none at all, was the result of the class aggression carried out by the Reagan and Bush administrations, with the support of the Democratic-controlled Congress, over the past thirteen years. The result—an unprecedented crisis in health care—has led to such an enormous demand for change that health care reform became the second most important issue (after jobs) in the 1992 election. Thirty-two percent of Bill Clinton's supporters voted for him because he endorsed health care reform, yet he has endorsed the corporate response to reform.[2] Chapter 3 discusses the impact of Clinton's election, the political and economic forces that are shaping his proposals, and the popular mobilization to change them.

The history of a society and its health care is the result not only of corporate class dominance, but of popular pressures for change. It is this conflict between and among classes that explains the changes that occur both in the society and its medicine. The working class and its instruments (trade unions and political parties) in the advanced capitalist countries have been the primary force behind the establishment of universal and comprehensive health benefits, which are in turn a key element of the welfare state. Chapter 4 shows how the type of financing and delivery of health services in the developed capitalist countries is the result of the combination of class forces in each society. It also shows how the absence of a national health program in the United States is related to the weakness of the working class and the absence of a political instrument that represents its interests.

An important and urgent political task is to change the knowledge, practice, and institutions of medicine to make them responsive to people's needs. This will not occur, however, without an active mobilization for change in U.S. society—a society in which the few rather than the many now control the major institutions, including the institutions of medicine. This will require breaking with the classism, racism, and sexism that dominate these institutions, which are discussed in Chapter 5.

These chapters are based on a series of lectures I gave to a student-sponsored forum on "Health, Medicine, and Society" at The Johns Hopkins University. They are written in nonacademic language to help people understand not so much *what* is wrong with the U.S. health care system—the majority of Americans already know this because they suffer from it—but *why* it is wrong. A whole academic and media industry exists to obfuscate rather than clarify this critical question. It is my hope that this book will help people to understand the root of their predicament and that from there they will go on to organize to change it.

I owe a note of recognition to the many people whom I have come to know during the years that I have been working on this topic. First and foremost to Mary McCormick, Anne Lorraine, and John Dunlop, and to the thousands of people like them that

I have met while trying to change the health sector in this country. Their heroic lives have been a constant source of inspiration. Also, thanks are owed to the many friends and colleagues involved in the current struggle to establish a single-payer health care system that, like the system in Canada, would provide comprehensive coverage to everyone. What I have learned as the result of my participation in this movement has enriched my intellectual work enormously. Such a relationship between theory and practice is of paramount importance not only for understanding our reality but for changing it as well. The former project is considerably weaker in the absence of the latter. A large body of academic work by progressive intellectuals is seriously impaired and impoverished by an ivory tower isolation that nurtures academism, narcissism, and irrelevance. There is an urgent need for progressive intellectuals to engage in political practice that can enrich their work and make it relevant to the lives of the working people of this country.

I also wish to thank my colleagues and students, with whom I have had many intensive and enjoyable discussions. If they were assisted by our exchanges as much as I was, I feel fully rewarded. Special thanks go to my friend David Himmelstein, who went through parts of the manuscript in great detail and provided much assistance.

I also owe a very particular debt of gratitude to two persons in my professional environment who helped me enormously in the preparation of the book. Linda Hansford, my technical editor, and Judith Bremmerman, my assistant, both provided invaluable assistance. Without them this book would not have been written. Thanks also to my good friends Paul Sweezy and Harry Magdoff, who were the first to encourage me to write the book and the most persistent in urging me to finish it. Susan Lowes, Director of Monthly Review Press, kept the pressure on. Finally, thanks to all those who will be working in the book's production, printing, and distribution.

1

WHY THE U.S. HEALTH CARE SYSTEM DOES NOT RESPOND TO PEOPLE'S NEEDS

Health care in the United States is in a state of profound crisis. In 1992 the United States spent $838 billion ($3,010 per person) on health services. No other country in the world spent such a large amount, which came to 14 percent of the Gross National Product, or GNP, almost double the average for capitalist countries with similar levels of economic development. Yet despite this high level of expenditure, 38 million Americans—17 percent of the population—have *no* health benefits, another 50 million have major gaps in their benefits, and the overwhelming majority do not have comprehensive coverage. If you or your parents, for example, were to develop a chronic condition that required

Figure 1-1
Growth of Uninsured Americans, 1976–1990

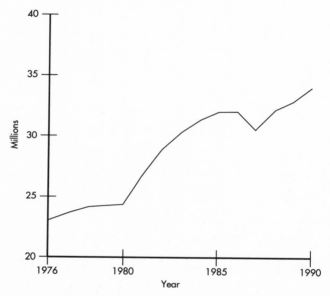

Detailed sources for all figures and tables will be found on pp. 119–120.

long-term care, you would probably be in deep trouble. The average annual cost for long-term care is $27,243, far more than a family earning the median income ($30,000) can afford. Not surprisingly, the inability to pay for health care is the primary cause of personal bankruptcy in this country. People are constantly denied care because they cannot pay their medical bills, or their health benefits are dropped because they cannot pay their health premiums or because they cost their employers or insurers too much. David Himmelstein and Steffie Woolhandler of Harvard University estimate that 100,000 people in the United States die

Figure 1-2
Who Are the Uninsured?

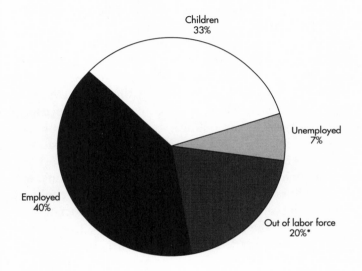

*Students under 18, homemakers, disabled, early retirees

each year from lack of care—three times as many as die from AIDS.

High costs and insufficient coverage are the key characteristics of the U.S. health care non-system, the most inefficient and inhuman of any health care system in any developed capitalist country. The United States and South Africa are the only major countries whose governments do not provide a national health program that guarantees access to health care in time of need. Health care in the United States is not a right; it is a privilege. At a time when the U.S. government declares that it is the great defender of human rights around the world, it continues to ignore this basic right at home. Forty years after the United Nations passed the Declaration of Human Rights, which in-cludes—among other things—the right to access to health care, the U.S. government does not guarantee a right that is guaranteed in most other developed countries. Why?

In order to understand this situation, we must look not only at the practice of medicine but at the society of which this practice is a component. In other words, in order to understand the tree—the health sector—we must study the forest—the society we live in. We therefore have to start our analysis by focusing on the social, economic, and political forces that shape our society and that also shape its health care, including its organization and its funding. This point cannot be overemphasized. Most expla-nations of our health care system describe the interactions among the various interest groups in the medical sector, including the insurance companies, the medical professional associations, the hospital lobbies, the drug companies, and so on. While these studies contain a great deal of valuable information, they do not fully explain why and how these groups operate, and with what consequences. Such studies miss the social and political contexts in which these groups interact. Yet it is the context that defines what is possible and not possible, what happens and what does not happen.

How can we go about understanding this context? This is a good question, and it has a complex answer.

First we need to understand power and how it is distributed. Power is very unevenly distributed. Most of us recognize, for example, that blacks, Hispanics, and other minorities in the United States have less power than whites, and that women have less power than men. Race and gender are categories of power, and much has been written about how racism and sexism con-tinue to operate in the society at large, as well as in its health care system.

But the United States is divided not only by race and gender, but also by *class*. Class is the most important category of power for understanding U.S. society and its system of medicine. Yet class is rarely discussed in either the scientific literature or the mainstream media. It is considered an almost "un-American" category. Yet in other countries, class is considered an extremely important category for understanding how people live, work, dress, vote, enjoy themselves, get sick, and die. In the United States, however, the category of class disappears: the majority of the population is supposed to be in the middle. It is accepted that there are extremes—the rich and the poor—but most Americans are believed to belong to the middle class. As former President George Bush once said, "Class is for European democracies or something else—it isn't for the United States of America. We are not going to be divided by class."[1]

But the United States does have classes. How people live, get sick, and die, as well as the type of health care that they receive, depends not only on their race and gender, but primarily on the class to which they belong. Furthermore, the majority of people know this. Among working people—those whose financial identity is determined by hourly wage rates—there is a profoundly felt sense of "them" (the bosses and their kind) and "us" (the workers). In spite of the mainstream press's constant repetition of the myth that we are a "middle-class" society, more people define themselves as working class than as middle class.[2] People contrast the powerful messages they receive through the media with another powerful set of messages that come from their daily experiences. What they believe is a synthesis of these contradictory messages. Every day they are told by the media that they belong to the middle class, but their daily reality does not match that image. That is why working people never simply repeat what those in power want them to believe.

Understanding the class structure of the United States and how it is reproduced over time is of enormous importance if we are to understand U.S. society and its health sector.

Figure 1-3
Occupational Distribution by Social Class and Gender, 1990

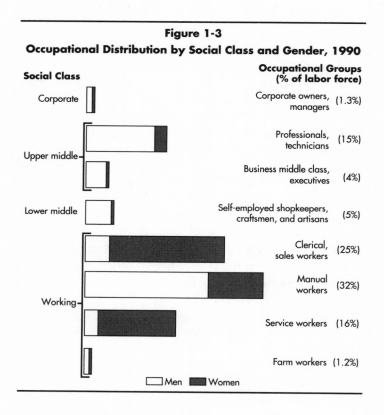

Social Class

Occupational Groups (% of labor force)

Corporate — Corporate owners, managers (1.3%)

Upper middle — Professionals, technicians (15%)

Business middle class, executives (4%)

Lower middle — Self-employed shopkeepers, craftsmen, and artisans (5%)

Working — Clerical, sales workers (25%)

Manual workers (32%)

Service workers (16%)

Farm workers (1.2%)

☐ Men ■ Women

THE U.S. CLASS STRUCTURE

Figure 1-3 shows the U.S. occupational and social class structure in 1990. At the top is a very small group (not more than 1.3 percent of the population) that has enormous power. This is what we can call the corporate class, and it includes individuals whose incomes come primarily from property rather than work. In Europe, this group is called the bourgeoisie. In the United States we do not use that term—it sounds too French—and instead call them the "very rich." Whatever name we use, the members of the corporate class hold a lot of power, including in the health care sector. This class is predominantly white and its leaders are predominantly male.

The next group is the middle class. Contrary to popular belief, the middle class does not constitute the majority of Americans, although it is much larger than the corporate class. It includes professionals, small businesspeople, self-employed shopkeepers, artisans, and so on.

The largest group is the working class, which includes almost 75 percent of the population. This is a class whose occupational structure and race and gender composition have changed over the past fifty years. The blue-collar sector of the working class—those working in heavy manufacturing—has declined, while the service sector has grown dramatically. The health sector is the fastest growing sector in the economy, and the health care industry is now the largest employer in the country. The total number of jobs in this sector increased by 639,000 from May 1990 through May 1992, while the total number of jobs *fell* by almost 1.8 million.

At the same time there has been a change from a predominantly white male working class to one in which women and minorities represent more than half of all wage earners. Changes in the labor force in the health care industry reflect the changes in the racial and gender make up of the working class as a whole. Today, most workers in the health sector are women, and 28 percent are minorities.

In the analysis of the U.S. class structure, we can see two striking phenomena that typify our society. One is the enormous concentration of wealth at the top. To cite just one statistic, the top 1 percent of the population, members of the corporate or capitalist class, owns 40 percent of all the property in this country, including stocks, bonds, and private land. While such an enormously skewed concentration of wealth is a characteristic of all capitalist societies, Figure 1-4 shows that it is more extreme in the United States.

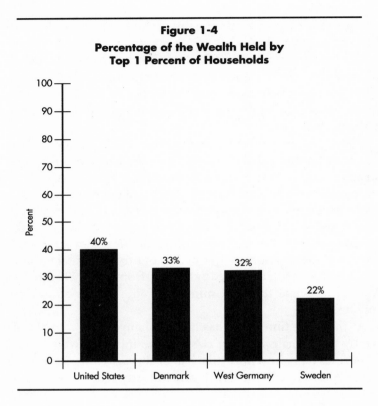

Figure 1-4
Percentage of the Wealth Held by
Top 1 Percent of Households

The other key characteristic of the U.S. class structure is the concentration of income at the top (see Figure 1-5). Nobel Prize winner Paul Samuelson, in his book *Economics*, wrote that "If we made today an income pyramid out of a child's blocks, with each layer portraying $1,000 of income, the peak would be far higher than the Eiffel Tower, but almost all of us would be within a yard of the ground."[3]

The social class structure is different in each of the three major sectors of the economy—the monopolistic sector, the competitive sector, and the state sector. Table 1-1 shows these three sectors and their production and labor force characteristics.

Figure 1-5

Average Income for Family Income Groups, 1992

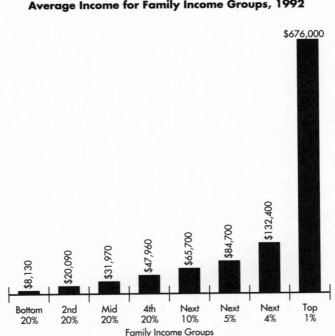

Of the three sectors, the monopolistic sector is the most influential. It includes the large financial and manufacturing companies and is the world of "corporate America"—the Fortune 500 companies and other large employers. This sector employs approximately 25 percent of the labor force. A few companies control each specific area of production or services. A key industry in this sector is the insurance industry, which plays, as we shall see, a very important role in the financing of health services.

The second sector, the market or competitive sector, used to be the largest of the three sectors in terms of both employment and economic activity, but it has declined over the past thirty

Table 1-1

Sectors of the U.S. Economy, with Production and Labor Force Characteristics

	State			Competitive
	Monopolistic	**Contractual**	**Public Service**	
Characteristics of Production	Primarily manufacturing		Primarily service	Primarily trade and service
	Economic concentration		Economic deconcentration	Economic deconcentration
	Highly monopolistic		Monopolistic	Competitive
	Vertical and horizontal integration (conglomerates)		Vertical and sectoral integration	Vertical and sectoral integration
	National and international		Federal, state, local	Regional and local
Characteristics of the Labor Force	Predominantly male		Predominantly female	Predominantly female
	Nonwhites: underrepresented		Nonwhites: proportionally represented	Nonwhites: overrepresented
	Unionized		Nonunionized	Nonunionized
	Salaries: relatively high		Salaries: medium	Salaries: low

years. This sector is generally labor intensive and local or regional in scope. The labor force is scattered in small units and seldom unionized. Examples are small businesses, restaurants, drug-stores, and, in the medical sector, fee-for-service solo or group practices.

The third major sector is the state (or government) sector, which is in turn divided into two subsectors. In the public service subsector, the government both funds and provides services—an example is the Public Health Service. It does this at all levels of government, federal, state, and local. The other subsector—the contractual subsector—includes those activities that the government funds but that are delivered by the private sector under contract. For the most part, the government contracts with the monopolistic sector—the defense industry is a prime example. The United States, unlike most developed capitalist countries, does not have a nationalized defense industry that produces armaments; instead the government contracts with large corporations for their manufacture. Two other examples of this type of contractual arrangement between the government and the private sector are Medicare (the federal program that funds health care for the elderly) and Medicaid (the federal program for the medically indigent). These, along with other federal and state health programs, make up 42 percent of all expenditures in the health sector. The government contracts with private service providers or with health insurance companies for the delivery of health care to the private sector. Most hospitals and physicians are private, and many of the facilities, equipment, drugs, and other commodities used in the health services are also produced and provided by private companies. As Table 1-2 shows, most of the major suppliers to the health sector are also major suppliers to the defense industry.

These corporations are major components of both the mili-tary-industrial and medical-industrial complexes. Other components of the medical-industrial complex, besides the medical and hospital equipment industries, are the insurance companies, the

Table 1-2

Major Manufacturing and Service Companies Operating in the Health Care Industry

Company	Fortune 500 Rank (1984)	Sales (billions $)	Major Areas of Production	Medical Production
IBM	6	45.0	Controls 60 percent U.S. computer, business typewriter, office equipment market	No. 1 in hospital computer market
General Electric	9	27.0	Consumer, industrial, military, technical systems; no. 6 contractor to Pentagon ($4.5 billion in sales); no. 2 producer of nuclear reactors	Diagnostic-imaging equipment; CAT scanners, X-ray, ultrasound, MRI
McDonnell-Douglas	34	9.5	Military and commercial aircraft; F-4 Phantom and F-15 Eagle; DC-9 and DC-10; computer and data-processing systems; no. 1 Pentagon defense contractor ($7.7 billion)	Health Services Division, formerly McAuto, fiscal intermediary for NYC Medicaid; acquired Science Dynamics Corp., renamed McDonnell-Douglas Physicians Systems, specializing in medical data bases and electronic claims-processing capabilities
Honeywell	56	6.0	Computer, information, and data systems in aerospace and defense; spacecraft; military and commercial aircraft; 10 percent of business with Pentagon	Controls 5 percent of hospital patient monitoring market; 1981 joint venture with NV Philips, manufacturing medical electronic systems
Siemens AG*	—	14.5	Germany's leading technology firm; world's third largest in telecommunications; supplying Brazil with 4 nuclear reactors	World's largest supplier of X-ray equipment and other diagnostic-imaging machinery
Avon Products	127	3.0	World's largest direct-selling business; cosmetics, toiletries, fragrances	Purchased Malinckrodt in 1982, producer of radiopharmaceuticals, X-ray contrast

*German-based multinational

drug companies, the hospitals, and the medical professional associations. These are the dominant power holders in the health sector. As we will see later, most debates over health policy have been internal discussions among components of this complex.

THE CORPORATE CLASS: THE MONOPOLISTIC SECTOR

Of the three sectors, the monopolistic sector is the most influential. It is called monopolistic because a few companies control most of the market in each of the commodities they produce. For example, the top computer company controls 60 percent of all computer sales; the top long-distance telephone company controls 70 percent of all such sales; the top airplane manufacturer controls 55 percent of all aircraft sales; the top four car manufacturers control 84 percent of all automobile sales—and so on. Put another way, the twenty largest manufacturing companies own a larger share of total manufacturing assets than the smallest 419,000 companies combined.

This enormous concentration of power is bad for democracy. The decisions made by these corporations have an enormous impact on the lives and well-being of millions of people who do not have any voice in those decisions. For example, when General Motors, the largest automobile manufacturer in the country, decided in 1991 to cut production by 12 percent, twenty-one plants were closed and 74,000 workers were laid off. Thousands and thousands of families and communities were hurt. Unemployment and the threat of unemployment mean death and disease. According to a report of the U.S. Congress, every 1 percent increase in unemployment leads to 5,000 deaths and 250,000 stress-related conditions. You might ask how a society that does not allow private ownership of atomic bombs because of the danger that this would entail nevertheless allows private ownership of corporations that can have similarly devastating consequences on the fabric of our society. The deterioration in the quality of life that has accompanied the decline of the high-wage sector of our economy is partially the result of decisions taken by corporate America to move its manufacturing plants to countries where labor is cheaper and there is less environmental regulation.

This situation has led to a growing interest in finding out who controls, or at least has a dominant influence in, the top corporations. According to a Congressional committee report, "The top hundred corporations control 65 percent of all corporate stocks in this country. And these top hundred corporations appear to be dominated by eight institutions, including six banks."[4] In other words, the top corporations are not self-sufficient in terms of financial capital. They depend on the financial institutions for their capital needs. This dependency means that financial institutions—particularly the large banks—have a huge influence on corporate policies through their ownership of corporate stocks and through interlocking directorships on their boards. The banks also have interlocking directorships with insurance companies, which are another important source of capital. Through the banks, the insurance companies exercise a major influence in corporate America. For example, of the 28 directors of Metropolitan Life Insurance, one of the largest insurance companies, 23 also sit on the boards of banking and related institutions, including Chase Manhattan Bank. Chase Manhattan in turn owns 10 percent of the stock of American Airlines, 8 percent of United Airlines, 15 percent of the Columbia Broadcasting System (CBS), 6 percent of Mobil Oil, and so on. Chase Manhattan and three other banks own 10 percent of International Telephone and Telegraph, 12 percent of Xerox, 22 percent of Gulf Oil, 10 percent of International Paper, 12 percent of Polaroid, and parts of many other powerful corporations. The House Banking and Currency Subcommittee once noted that ownership of 5 percent of a corporation's stock is sufficient to give the owners a controlling vote in that corporation.[5]

The insurance companies and the banking industry therefore have an enormous influence on our economic and social life. Yet none of the people who sit on the boards of these institutions has been elected and none is accountable to the public, although their decisions often dominate our lives. The power of these companies is symbolized by their domination of the skylines of many of our cities. In Boston, for instance, the two tallest buildings are the headquarters of major insurance companies—the John Hancock Tower and the Prudential Center. Like the cathedrals of the Middle Ages, they represent the center of power in the urban landscape.

THE INSURANCE INDUSTRY IN THE HEALTH SECTOR

Insurance companies (such as Prudential and John Hancock) write more than 50 percent of the health insurance premiums in this country. They are referred to in the health sector as the *commercial health insurance companies* to distinguish them from the *voluntary health insurance companies,* or the Blues, which until the 1960s controlled most of the premiums. The Blues' share of the private health insurance market dropped from 45 percent in 1965 to 33 percent in 1986, and it continues to decline.

The Blues were established during the Depression of the 1930s by the hospitals (which established Blue Cross) and the American Medical Association (which established Blue Shield) in order to ensure that hospitals and physicians would not run out of patients. For an annual payment—called a premium—these two groups promised to cover many, although not all, of the health care needs of those they insured. Working people could afford to pay a fixed (and at that time, small) amount of money for premiums but could not afford to pay doctors' fees for every service they needed. Later on, after the Depression, the price of premiums increased considerably, but the system of prepayment remained. Blue Cross has continued to be the insurance instrument of the hospital industry and Blue Shield of the medical profession.

Blue Cross pays the hospitals for their "reasonable" costs,

leaving the hospitals to define what is reasonable. Blue Shield pays physicians according to "usual and customary" fees; if these are not too far from the fees of other physicians in the area, Blue Shield will pay. Such a generous physician reimbursement policy does not exist anywhere else in the world.

The Blues were given tax exempt status in return for their agreement to offer coverage based on an average premium for the community in which they operated, rather than requiring sicker people to pay higher premiums and healthy people to pay lower premiums. But once the commercial insurance companies began to enter the health premium market, the Blues were forced to compete for customers. This forced them to choose only customers who would be "good risks"—healthy people who would not need expensive care. Before long both the Blues and the commercial insurers were avoiding the sick and vulnerable and favoring the young and healthy. In 1986, Congress, recognizing this development, withdrew the Blues' tax exemption.

There is a great deal of competition between the Blues and the commercial insurance companies over control of the premium market. The commercials have been winning the battle, since the insurance companies have far more economic and political influence than the Blues. The large commercial insurance companies are not just health insurers—health is but one piece of their business. Their assets are enormous: Prudential has $116 billion in assets; Metropolitan Life, $94 billion; Aetna, $49 billion; Connecticut General, $31 billion; Travellers, $30 billion; and so on. The boards of directors of the insurance companies are filled with the world's wealthiest people. To take only one example, James Lynn, chief executive officer of Aetna, earned an astounding $23 million in 1990. In 1992, President Clinton's candidate for attorney general, Zoë Baird, made $1.5 million as a vice-president of Aetna.

Today, more and more physicians work for insurance-controlled medical conglomerates, forcing the loss of their professional autonomy. The invasion of corporate capitalist relationships into medicine has meant, as the great social thinkers Karl Marx and Friedrich Engels predicted, that "the bourgeoisie has stripped of its halo every occupation hitherto honored and looked up to with reverent awe. It has converted the physician, the lawyer, the priest, the poet, the man [and woman] of science, into its paid wage laborers."[6] Although Marx and Engels may have overstated the case, since physicians certainly do not become members of the working class, the loss of professional autonomy is nevertheless a very much resented reality, as most physicians who work for the conglomerates will tell you. The mountains of paperwork, the supervision, and the administrative interference in clinical decisions are some of the most frequent areas of complaint.

The dominance of the insurance companies in the health care sector has meant that they, rather than the providers of care, are the ones who have a commanding voice in that sector. As a result, it is frequently not physicians and other health professionals who decide what their patients need; it is the insurance companies. What many people do not realize is that any procedures a physician recommends must be approved by the patient's insurance company. A physician can spend up to an hour a day seeking permission to do what he or she considers best for the patient. The insurance companies base their decision on their own criteria of cost-effectiveness, which are not disclosed to either the patient or the physician. This degree of intrusion into the physician-patient relationship by a third party—the insurance company—is unheard of in other countries.

THE POWER OF THE INSURANCE INDUSTRY

In the United States, economic power means political power. The corporate class that controls the insurance companies has enormous political power. It exercises this power in many different ways. One is by funding members of Congress who sit on the committees that write health legislation. From 1981 to the first half of 1991, for instance, the insurance industry's political action committees (or PACs) contributed $60 million to members of Congress, with much of the money going to the chairs and key members of health-related committees. This included some of the leading "liberals" in both the Senate and the House, such as Congressman Pete Stark, Senator Bill Bradley, Senator Jay Rockefeller, and Senator Tom Harkin, among many others. These same people also received $28 million from the medical-professional PACs, $9 million from the pharmaceutical PACs, and $6 million from the hospital PACs. Of the twenty-one senators who received more than $200,000 from medical-industry PACs, twelve serve on the Senate Finance Committee, which makes decisions about Medicare and other health-related matters. The twenty-five representatives who have received the greatest amounts of medical-industry PAC money all hold leadership positions in the House or are members of the Ways and Means or Energy and Commerce committees. For instance, Democratic Representative Pete Stark, chair of the House Ways and Means health subcommittee, has received money from almost all the health-related PACs. Senator David Durenberger, the ranking Republican on the Senate's Medicare subcommittee, is the favorite recipient of contributions from hospital industry PACs. Former Senate Finance Committee chair (and now Secretary of the Treasury in the Clinton administration) Democrat Lloyd Bentsen received substantial amounts of money from the insurance industry. Senator Max Baucus, a high-ranking member of the Senate Finance Committee and also a Democrat, has been generously supported by physicians and insurance companies. And another Democrat, Representative Henry Waxman, chair of the Energy and Commerce health subcommittee, has received money from the American Medical Association and other medical groups. Stark, Waxman, and Bentsen have introduced legislative proposals that have been heavily influenced by their sponsors.[7] As Senator Barbara Mikulski has noted, we have the best Congress money can buy.

Some industries and PACs also give generously to both the Democratic and Republican parties. In 1991, Aetna, Warner-

Lambert, Chubb, the American Dental Association's PAC, and the Humana hospital chain each gave so-called "soft money" contributions of $20,000 to the Republican Party. Blue Cross and Blue Shield gave $29,000 to the Republicans and almost $17,000 to the Democrats. Upjohn gave $25,000 to the Democrats and $23,000 to the Republicans. And Glaxo, another drug company, gave $50,000 to the Democrats. Table 1-3 shows PAC contributions from the health industry during the 1992 elections.

The result of this corrupting situation is a substantial reduction of the democratic process. Let me share with you one example of what I mean. The insurance companies—the commercials and the Blues—as well as the other components of the medical-industrial complex, such as the medical-provider lobbies, the hospital lobbies, the equipment and pharmaceutical lobbies, among others, are the main forces responsible for the fact that the United States is the only major capitalist country without a national health program that guarantees universal and comprehensive health benefits to our population. The overwhelming majority of the population is dissatisfied with health care in this country, and 82 percent wants major and profound changes in the system of funding health care.[8] By a majority or large plurality, Americans since 1952—when the Gallup polls first asked this question— have wanted the federal government to finance health care. But they still do not have it. Back in the 1970s, the labor unions and their allies in Congress—Senator Edward Kennedy and Congresswoman Martha Griffiths—put forward a proposal for a national health program that would cover everyone and would be financed by the federal government, which would then contract directly with the providers of health services (as is done in Canada). The government would be the *single payer for health services,* eliminating the insurance companies. Needless to say, the insurance lobbies and their close friends in Congress mobilized to stop that proposal.

And they succeeded. The Kennedy-Griffiths bill was redesigned and reintroduced as the Kennedy-Mills bill. Congressman

Table 1-3
Major PAC Contributors

**Political action committees that contributed the most money
to candidates in the 1992 election**

National Association of Realtors	$2,950,138
American Medical Association	2,936,086
International Brotherhood of Teamsters	2,442,552
Association of Trial Lawyers of America	2,336,135
National Education Association	2,323,122

**Political action committees in the health industry that contributed
the most money to candidates in the 1992 election**

American Medical Association	$2,936,086
American Dental Association	1,420,958
American Academy of Ophthalmology	801,527
American Chiropractic Association	641,746
American Hospital Association	505,888
American Podiatry Association	401,000
American Optometric Association	398,366
American Health Care Association	382,019
American College of Emergency Physicians	330,725
American Nurses Association	306,519
Association for the Advancement of Psychology	273,743
American Physical Therapy Association	198,941
Eli Lilly & Company	195,530
Pfizer Inc.	188,100
Schering-Plough Corporation	186,050

Wilbur Mills was the chair of the powerful House Ways and
Means Committee and was very close to the insurance industry—
and also close to a stripper. The latter connection, not the former,
created a scandal and Mills had to resign two years later. He was
found with the stripper in a compromising position. Mills had,
however, been in a compromising position with the insurance
companies for a long time. The Kennedy-Mills bill put the insur-

ance companies back on the scene. They were to continue to be in charge of the funding and administration of health insurance. As the *New York Times* editorialized, the decision "to retain the insurance companies' role was based on recognition of that industry's power to kill any legislation it considers unacceptable. The bill's sponsors thus had to choose between appeasing the insurance industry and obtaining no national health insurance at all."[9] But even with the changes made to appease the industry, the Kennedy-Mills bill was defeated. The status quo won.

We also saw the enormous political influence of the insurance companies during the 1992 election campaign. Even though the majority of Americans would prefer a health system like the Canadian one, not one of the candidates dared to propose it, afraid of antagonizing the insurance industry and the medical-industrial complex. Even Tom Harkin, considered one of the most liberal members of the Senate, remained silent about the need to establish a national health program, emphasizing instead—as a cop out—the need to improve our "preventive services." Harkin received $270,404 from the medical-insurance PACs, which may explain his deafening silence on one of the major topics of the campaign. Similarly, the directors of the health components of both the Bush and Clinton campaigns were Washington lobbyists for the insurance companies. The Republican's chief health advisor was Deborah Steelman, a lobbyist representing the Pharmaceutical Manufacturers Association, Aetna Life and Casualty, and others. The Democrat's chief health advisor was Bruce Fried, also a lobbyist for the major health insurance companies.

The corrupting influence of corporate America over the political process is encouraged by the "revolving door"—the movement of former politicians and the staff of the major health-related congressional committees to jobs in the medical-industrial complex. The majority of Washington lobbyists for the medical-industrial complex once worked in the Congress and have retained close contacts there. The following (compiled by

Common Cause in March 1992) will give an idea of the extent of this process:

Frank McLaughlin
- *Then:* Aide to former House Speaker Tip O'Neill
- *Now:* Head of the American Dental Association's PAC

John Salmon
- *Then:* Aide to House Ways and Means Committee Chair Dan Rostenkowski
- *Now:* Lobbies for the Federation of American Health Systems

Kenneth Bowler
- *Then:* Staff director of the House Committee on Ways and Means
- *Now:* Lobbies for Pfizer

John Jonas
- *Then:* Tax counsel for the House Committee on Ways and Means
- *Now:* Lobbies for Metropolitan Life, Massachusetts Mutual Life, and the National Association of Life Underwriters

Richard Verville
- *Then:* Assistant secretary of Health, Education, and Welfare
- *Now:* Lobbies for the Academy of Physical Medicine and Rehabilitation, Medical Group Management, and the Joint Council on Allergy and Immunology

Dawson Mathis
- *Then:* Member of Congress
- *Now:* Lobbies for Metropolitan Life and Massachusetts Mutual Life

Gordon Wheeler
- *Then:* Congressional liaison, Office of Management and the Budget; assistant to President Bush
- *Now:* Political affairs director, Health Insurance Association of America

Deborah Steelman
- *Then:* Domestic policy adviser to Bush transition team; Office of Management and the Budget official
- *Now:* Medical industry lobbyist

Martin Gold
- *Then:* Counsel to former Senate Majority Leader Howard Baker
- *Now:* Lobbies for the American Medical Association and the College of American Pathologists

And there is more: former President Ronald Reagan used to work for the American Medical Association and opposed the establishment of Medicare. In a phonograph record sent by the AMA to doctors' wives, Reagan warned: "If you and I don't stop Medicare we will spend our sunset years telling our children and children's children what it was like in America when men were free."[10] Both former President Bush and former Vice-President Dan Quayle used to work for the pharmaceutical industry.

The U.S. Constitution starts with that splendid sentence, "We, the People..." To be accurate, we should add a footnote that would read "and the medical-industrial complex." The latter has a far greater voice than the people in deciding what can and cannot be done in the health sector.

CLASS CONTROL OF THE HEALTH CARE INSTITUTIONS

The corporate class's control over the health care sector does not begin and end with its control of funding; it continues with control over the health care institutions themselves and over the political institutions that influence how these work. Money, the energy that moves the system, passes through institutional channels that are controlled, or heavily influenced, by groups that are similar, although not identical, to those that have dominant influence in the funding of those institutions.

Who controls the health care institutions, such as the medical research foundations, teaching hospitals, voluntary hospitals, and others? The question is difficult to answer. There are many groups that shape these institutions, but one that has enormous power is the board of directors (or trustees, or executive board) of each institution. These boards not only set policy, but generally appoint the executive officers and many members of upper level management in these institutions. Listen to Abraham Flexner, author of the famous *Flexner Report,* which established medical education in the United States as we know it today. Flexner wrote that "the influence of the board of trustees of the university determines in the social and economic realms an atmosphere of timidity, which is not without effect on critical appointments and promotions."[11] Feminists have long been aware of this point and have rightly called for a change in the gender composition of the boards of directors of our health institutions. Blacks, Hispanics, and other minorities have been equally aware of the problems of having all-white boards and have demanded a change in their racial and ethnic composition so that they will better reflect the diversity of the communities they serve.

But the issue of the class composition of these boards is seldom raised. Figure 1-6 compares the class composition of the United States as a whole with the class composition of the boards of trustees of the top ten medical research foundations, the private medical teaching institutions, the state medical teaching institutions, and the voluntary hospitals.

The table shows vividly the enormous overrepresentation of the corporate and upper middle classes and the dramatic underrepresentation of the majority of the population—members of the lower middle and working classes. Further, the small changes in the gender and racial/ethnic composition of these boards have not had much effect on their class composition. Only in the case of the voluntary not-for-profit hospitals do members of the working class appear on these boards. As R. M. MacIver has written, "The typical board member is associated with large-scale business, a banker, a manufacturer, business executive or prominent lawyer."[12]

You could say—and it has often been said—that there is a justifiable explanation for the class control of these institutions: members of the corporate class are needed to raise funds for the

Figure 1-6
Social Class and Gender Composition of U.S. Labor Force, Health Labor Force, and Boards of Trustees in the Health Sector

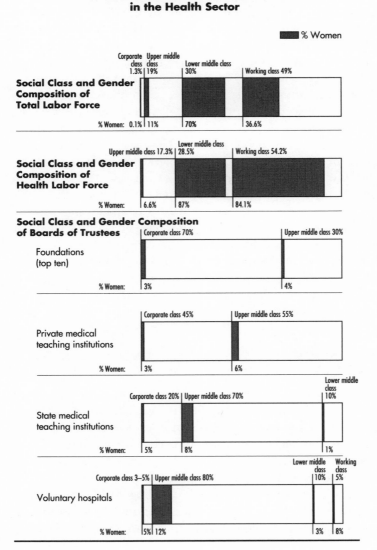

institution. But while that may have been the case in the past, it is not anymore. Most of the funding of the leading private teaching institutions is overwhelmingly public—in other words, the funds come from the majority of the American people, ordinary folks who are not represented on the boards of directors.

This class discrimination is not only the least recognized type of discrimination in the United States, but it is the most persistent and continuous form of discrimination. For example, Figure 1-7 shows the evolution of the class, race, and gender composition of U.S. medical students from 1920, when the *Flexner Report* was published and medical education was established, until 1992.

You can see that there has been an improvement in the representation of women and African-Americans in the medical student body. Although these changes are too timid, at least something is being done to correct this discrimination. But notice that the strongest, most persistent, and unchangeable form of discrimination is class discrimination (see Figure 1-7). In 1920, only 12 percent of all medical students came from families at or below the median family income—that is, in the lower economic half of the population. This percentage remained the same in 1992, seventy years later. This is a discrimination that very few people talk about.

THE CONSEQUENCES OF THE CLASS DOMINANCE OF OUR HEALTH CARE INSTITUTIONS

Why is the class dominance of our health care institutions worrisome? For many reasons. One reason, of particular importance in teaching institutions, is that it leads to the exclusion of positions that may deviate from or even confront the pattern of class positions. The pattern of class dominance in the health care institutions favors a climate of conformism and discourages the presentation of alternative views, including views that question the pattern of class dominance itself and the economic system that produces and maintains it. As economist John Kenneth

Figure 1-7
Changes in the Race, Class, and Gender Composition of the U.S. Population and of U.S. Medical Students

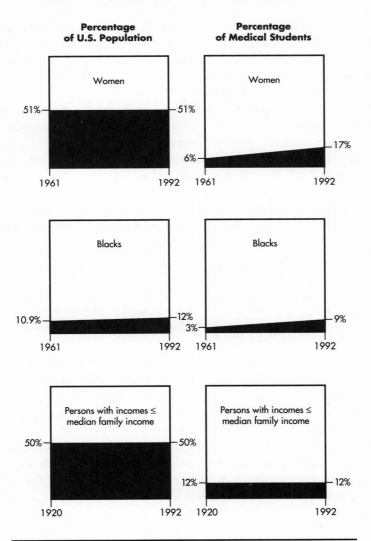

Galbraith once wrote, "Higher education is, of course, extensively accommodated to the needs of the industrial corporate system"[13]—or the private enterprise system in which the corporate class is dominant. His words were echoed by the then-president of Harvard University, Dr. Nathaniel Pusey, in a straightforward ideological statement: "The university as a whole ... is completely directed toward making the private enterprise system continue to work effectively and beneficially in a very difficult world."[14] How does that position fit with Harvard's lofty motto, "In Looking for Truth," unless it is assumed that the truth resides in the private enterprise system? Official and rhetorical statements aside, however, the primary function and purpose of one class dominating an institution's board of trustees is to perpetuate the values that will benefit their class and its interests. Other views, if they are allowed at all, are marginalized and those who hold them are deprived of the resources that would allow them to carry weight in the debate. As political scientist Ralph Miliband has written, the dominant value-generating systems

> contribute to the fostering of a climate of conformity, not by the total suppression of dissent, but by the presentation of views which fall outside the consensus as curious heresies, or, even more effectively, by treating them as irrelevant eccentricities, which serious and reasonable people may dismiss as of no consequence. This is very functional for the system.[15]

One example of the negative consequences of class discrimination in medicine is the very minor role given to occupational medicine, as well as to issues of occupational health and safety, in the curricula of medical schools and even of schools of public health. In fact, you can read through an entire medical school curriculum without even noticing that the majority of Americans are members of the working class. Occupational medicine is one of the least prestigious specialties, and many of its practitioners are forced to work for employers who hire and fire them according to the employers', rather than the employees', needs and interests.

Another negative consequence of class discrimination is the lack of, or limited, tenure in academic institutions of professors with anti-corporate views. An example from The Johns Hopkins University, where I teach, is the marginalization in the 1950s of the nation's greatest historian of medicine, Dr. Henry Sigerist. Because of his views, which were perceived as threatening to the corporate class, Sigerist was marginalized within the academic community and he finally left both Hopkins and the country. Although the situation is no longer so extreme, it is still the case that anti-corporate views are discriminated against in U.S. medical and health institutions.

CLASS POWER AND THE STATE IN THE HEALTH SECTOR

Having described the patterns of class dominance over the financing of health care and the administration of health care institutions, let me now touch on a third component of what is going on in the health care sector. This is the class influence on the government, including its executive, legislative, and judicial branches. According to official rhetoric, the U.S. government represents the voice of the people. As one widely used textbook put it, "In our nation, political power reflects the will of all people, not the will of a few at the top."[16]

The reality, however, is otherwise. Figure 1-8 compares the class composition of the country with the class composition of the cabinet, the Senate, and the House of Representatives. The data for elected officials reflect their class position before being elected. For example, Senator Barbara Mikulski of Maryland is counted as lower middle class because she was a social worker before she was elected. She is in a minority in the Senate: as you can see, the overwhelming majority of senators are members of the corporate and upper middle classes. The same applies to the cabinet. Business was the largest single occupational group in cabinet positions from 1989 to 1990: of all the cabinet members during this period, more than 80 percent had been in business of

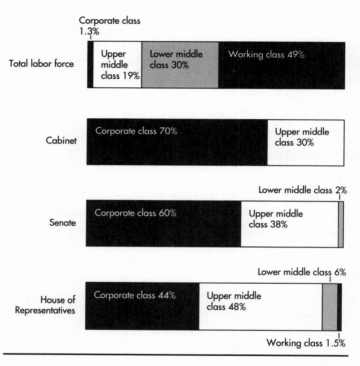

Figure 1-8

**Social Class Composition of the U.S. Labor Force
and of the Executive and Legislative Branches
of the Federal Government**

one sort or another. This situation persists in President Clinton's cabinet. In spite of Clinton's populist message, sustained throughout his presidential campaign, seven of his cabinet members are lawyers with close ties to corporate America. All seven made more than $1 million before being appointed.

The same pattern of class domination holds for the House. A total of 102 congresspeople held stock and well-paying executive positions in banks or other financial institutions, and 81 received regular income from law firms that generally represented big business. Sixty-three percent got income from stock in the top defense contractors; 45 percent from the giant (and federally regulated) oil and gas industries; 22 percent from radio and television companies; 11 percent from commercial airlines and 9 percent from railroads. Ninety-eight congresspeople were involved in numerous capital gains transactions.

This class bias is also evident in the federal health establishment. For instance, twelve of the last eighteen Secretaries of Health and Human Services had business backgrounds. At the other end of the social spectrum, however, labor representatives have filled few key positions in either the executive or legislative branches.

It is important to note that while much has been written about the limited representation of women, and of blacks and other minorities, in top political positions, almost nothing has been written about the very limited class representation in these same bodies.

Some might argue that while there is indeed a pattern of class domination in our major political institutions, they are still representative because these politicians were elected by the majority of citizens, who are, as we saw earlier, mostly working class. The problem with this argument is that the majority of the working class does not vote. People are fully aware of the enormous power that corporate America has over their political institutions: 72 percent, according to a recent *New York Times* poll, believe that the Congress represents powerful economic interests rather than ordinary people.[17] In fact, barely half of the population of voting age goes to the polls in presidential-year Congressional elections (52 percent in 1988 and 54 percent in 1992) and less than half in non-presidential-year Congressional elections (38 percent in 1990). Since the half that votes is predominantly the upper economic half, we can conclude that the lower half, which includes the majority of the working class, does not vote. Table 1-4 shows the correlation between income and

Table 1-4
**Relationship Between Income and Voter
Participation in Presidential Elections,
1984 and 1988 (average)**

Income	Percent Voting
$15,000 or less	32%
$15,000–$30,000	49%
$30,000–$40,000	56%
$40,000–$50,000	72%

voter participation: the lower the income, the lower the participation. The majority of working-class Americans do not vote
because they do not trust our political institutions. They do not
consider these institutions representative or responsive to their
interests. And they are right.

DIVERSITY WITHIN THE DOMINANT CLASSES
AND THE HEALTH POLICY DEBATE

There is, however, a diversity of interests within the dominant
classes, a diversity that is evident in the proposals for reforming
the health care system put forward by different groups. For
example, large financial capital (such as the major insurance
companies) has different interests than manufacturing companies or medical practitioners (as represented by the AMA). These
differences cause conflict. It is these conflicts between different
corporate interest groups that are at the center of the debate on
health care reform. The large insurance companies support the
"managed competition" model, a solution first put forward by
Alain Enthoven (former deputy director of defense under Robert
McNamara when he was directing the Vietnam war and later
health advisor to Prime Minister Margaret Thatcher on her plan
to privatize the National Health Service in Great Britain). Ac-

cording to the managed competition proposal, which is supported by the insurance companies, the AMA, the *New York Times*, and the Clinton-Gore administration, employees would have to enroll in insurance-operated health care plans chosen for them by their employers. The employees could expect to see their choice of providers, and their benefits, dramatically reduced.

A few corporate leaders, however, including those in such industries as automobile manufacturing, want the government to play a direct role in controlling the costs because these have become so high. For instance, employee health benefits are a larger component of the cost of a car than the steel it is built from: $700 of the cost of a car now goes to pay for health benefits, compared to only $200 in Canada or Japan. Further, large employers have come to realize that the growing cost of health insurance is cutting into company profits, at least in the short term. In the long term, of course, they can pass these costs on to workers by cutting wages. In fact, the growth in the cost of health benefits is the primary reason wages in the United States have remained constant since 1972. As noted by the Congressional Budget Office, "Since 1973, the increased costs for health care and other benefits have absorbed most of the gains in inflation-adjusted compensation, leaving little room for wages and salaries."[18]

Conflicts between workers and employers over health benefits were the primary cause of strikes in 1991 and 1992. This situation led large employers to provide their own health insurance rather than contracting out to the insurance companies. Today 60 percent of all employers self-insure their employees. This means that they have health insurance departments that administer health care benefits in order to control costs directly—rather than indirectly through the insurance companies. These employers were primarily responsible for the ERISA law, which allows an employer to curtail, reduce, or even eliminate health benefits for any employee who, because of a chronic condition such as AIDS, has health care costs that the employer considers too excessive for it to sustain. What this means is that an employee whose employer is self-insured has no medical security. This situation, recognized as legal by the Supreme Court, faces millions of workers who think that they have benefits until the moment they really need them—at which point they are dropped from their employers' health plan. Capitalism in the United States is a rough, cruel capitalism, a capitalism without gloves. You can see that there is a diversity of interests within the dominant classes in which insurance companies have different interests from large employers, which, in turn, have different interests from the medical trade and professional associations.

Despite the diversity of proposals for health care reform, there is a bias in the system that explains why some proposals have a far better chance than others, depending on whether or not they conflict with the structure of power that sustains the interests of the various groups. As one perceptive observer has written, the "flaw in the pluralist heaven is that the heavenly chorus sings with a very special accent ... the system is askew, loaded and unbalanced in favor of a fraction of a minority."[19] The political debate that reflects this pluralism takes place within the framework of a common understanding and acceptance of certain premises and assumptions that consistently benefit some classes rather than others.

Even though a large plurality or a majority of people have, since 1952, wanted a health care sytem in which the health services are allocated according to need rather than ability to pay, none of the proposals put forward by the White House or by the congressional leadership has even come close to suggesting such a system. This is a clear sign of class dominance.

THE ORIGINS OF EMPLOYMENT-BASED HEALTH COVERAGE

Understanding class dominance is of paramount importance not only for understanding why the United States does not have a national health plan, but also for understanding why health benefits are provided through the workplace. In 1989, for instance, 56.9 percent of workers received health benefits through their jobs. Why? To answer this question, we must go back to the late 1940s and early 1950s, the period after World War II. The U.S. working class made enormous sacrifices during World War II. It was a war against fascism and nazism, a war for a better future for working people and their children. Not surprisingly, then, at the end of the war people's expectations were high: they believed that their sacrifices had to have served a purpose. Powerful groups were asking for a redistribution of wealth, for the nationalization of banking, and for the establishment of a national health program run by the government. Working people were pushing for these demands, demands that threatened the capitalist and upper middle classes. In response to this threat, these classes developed an aggressive anti-working-class campaign. Congress, where the dominant classes had enormous influence, led the fight. The targets included progressive individuals in all areas of political, social, and academic life. That campaign—called McCarthyism—was brutal. (It was at that time that Henry Sigerist was forced to retire from teaching.)

In 1947, Congress passed the Taft-Hartley Act, which—among other things—outlawed sympathy strikes: for instance, coal miners could not go out on strike in support of steel workers. (For more on the act, see Chapter 5.) In other words, class pressure was outlawed. In no other Western developed capitalist country do workers face such restrictions. Indeed, it is not unusual to see a whole city—or even a whole country—in Europe paralyzed by a general strike, in which *all* the workers go on strike in support of demands that would benefit the majority of workers and their families. In the United States, a general strike is forbidden.

The Taft-Hartley Act also mandated that workers and their unions obtain health benefits from their employers through the collective bargaining process rather than, as in Europe, through the state. In other words, the unions had to negotiate the employers' payment of health insurance premiums for the workers and their families. This has meant that workers and their unions have to pressure their employers to get or to extend health benefits. Needless to say, wherever unions are strong, health benefits are extensive; where they are weak—as they are in most sectors of the economy—health benefits are limited.

The United States is therefore the only country in the developed world where workers and their families lose their health benefits when they lose their jobs. Relating health benefits to employment is an enormously effective way to discipline labor. Even changing jobs may mean changing the level of health benefits. According to a *New York Times*/CBS poll conducted in August 1991, 32 percent of working people stayed in jobs they did not like for fear of losing their health benefits.[20] The current shift from high-wage to low-wage, from union to non-union, and from full-time to part-time jobs has also meant a shift from good health benefits (in high-wage, unionized, and full-time jobs) to poor or nonexistent coverage (in low-wage, non-unionized, and part-time jobs). This shift was particularly large in the 1980s, during the Reagan/Bush years, when class aggression against the working class intensified. In 1979, 14.6 percent of the population (or 28.4 million people) did not have *any* form of health benefits. By 1985, this number had grown to 17.5 percent (36.8 million people). The majority were workers and their children. Thirteen percent of all full-time workers are uninsured. Most work for small employers who do not want, or cannot afford, to pay health benefits for their employees. Only 39 percent of small firms (those with twenty-five or less employees) offer health insurance to their workers, compared with 99 percent of firms with one hundred or more employees.

The same *New York Times*/CBS poll showed that 44.7 percent of those who change jobs or whose employment is for some reason interrupted did not have any form of health benefits for up to twenty-eight months. This percentage was even higher for blacks and Hispanics, who tend to be concentrated in low-wage nonunion jobs. Twenty percent of African-Americans and 33 percent of Hispanics are uninsured. Millions of people have loved ones who are sick and are not able to do anything about it because they cannot afford medical care.

But the problem does not end there. Compounding this inhuman situation is the huge reduction in benefits for working people that occurred during the 1980s. There was an almost 50 percent reduction in the hourly benefits (in dollar amounts) paid by employers for health insurance from 1980 to 1989 (from $1.63 per hour in 1980 to $0.85 in 1989), which led to a significant reduction in health care benefits for the majority of working people. In other words, during the 1980s, workers were not only growing more afraid of losing their jobs, and thus their health coverage, but even those who kept their jobs saw their benefits significantly reduced. This was the direct result of linking health care benefits to employment, and it is the situation that is favored by most large employers. In a recent survey of chief executive officers of Fortune 500 companies, the majority opposed the establishment of a national health program, preferring to continue employer-based coverage. They also opposed government assistance in providing health benefits to the unemployed, in order to scare workers into holding onto jobs that have deteriorating levels of wages and benefits. This is the political project of those who, like former President Bush, deny the existence of classes and class struggle in the United States and claim to believe in a "gentler America."

All these realities are the result of class power—the power of the dominant class—which is a power unparalleled in any other major capitalist country. Let me give you an example of how unparalleled that power is. We recently saw how Prime Minister Margaret Thatcher had to resign because of her growing unpopularity, which was largely due to the imposition of what the British call a poll tax. According to Thatcher's proposal, local services were to be financed by a flat tax on each household, so that rich households and working-class households would both pay the same amount. The Labour Party loudly denounced the poll tax and mobilized so much opposition that Thatcher was forced out of office.

Yet in this country most of us are forced to pay for health care according to a system that is not unlike the poll tax: every employee in a particular business or industry pays the same amount (we call it a premium rather than a poll tax) for their health benefits, regardless of income. Thus the chairman of Bethlehem Steel, whose annual salary is $1.2 million, pays approximately the same premium for himself and his family as does the unskilled black or white steelworker in one of his mills, in spite of the fact that his income is forty times larger. And it is the Democratic Party that is leading the way in expanding rather than changing this profoundly regressive way of funding health care. The Democratic leadership in the Congress is asking for the same thing that President Nixon asked for in 1974: the expansion of health benefits by mandating that small employers provide such coverage. Both Nixon in the 1970s and the leading forces in the Democratic Party in the 1990s are reacting to popular pressure to establish a national health program funded through general taxation. As Democratic Senator Jay Rockefeller, chairman of an influential congressional commission on health care, recently noted, "Employer-mandated coverage is the last resort we have against the establishment of a national health program that neither you nor I want."[21] He was talking to the major trade association of for-profit hospitals.

In the United Kingdom, as well as in all the other developed capitalist countries, workers have fought to divorce health benefits from the job and to make the funding of benefits progressive. This is why the overwhelming majority of the labor movements in the Western world made access to health care a universal entitlement, with the government guaranteeing that such a human right is implemented. Part of this human right is the funding of benefits through progressive taxation. In the United States, both the Republican and the Democratic parties have been proponents of the regressive funding of health services.

2

CLASS STRUGGLE IN THE HEALTH SECTOR DURING THE REAGAN/BUSH YEARS

In reading the newspapers, watching television news, or listening to the radio during the past thirteen years, we witnessed several events that had a profound effect on the health of Americans. On the one hand, we saw a substantial increase in military expenditure, a growth that took place in a political climate that can best be described as "war hysteria," in which even the unthinkable—a nuclear war—became part of normal political discourse. During the 1980s, not only military leaders but also political and academic leaders spoke of the possibility of "limited" nuclear war. In February 1983, Eugene Rostow, an advisor to the Reagan administration, reminded Americans that the Soviet Union remained a major power even after losing 20 million people during World War II. By the same token, he argued, the United States could survive a similar loss and still remain a major force in the world.[1] This type of talk created a climate in which, according to a 1984 Gallup poll, 50 percent of young Americans believed that there would be a nuclear war in the coming decade.[2] In the ten years from 1980 to 1990, the government spent $2 *trillion* on the military, more than was spent during the thirty previous years. On the other hand, during the past thirteen years we also saw substantial cuts in federal expenditures on health and social services. Health centers were closed, school budgets cut, many health programs discontinued, and government regulations to protect workers, consumers, and the environment were weakened or dismantled.

It must be stressed that these policies were bipartisan: they were approved by the Republican administration and the Democratic-controlled Congress and supported by both political parties. In fact, the unprecedented (in peacetime) increase in military expenditures and the equally unprecedented decline in health and social expenditures were both initiated by President Jimmy Carter. Edward Snyder, of the Friends Committee on National Legislation, described Carter's 1979 budget as follows:

> What we see in this budget is, an additional $89 million for the Army XM-1 tank program; mental health centers cut $88 million.
> An additional $141 million for A-10 attack aircraft; cancer research cut $55 million.
> An additional $719 million for nuclear attack submarines; food stamp program cut $865 million.[3]

Snyder went on and on, detailing the transfer of federal funds from the social sector to the military. A year later, on December 10, 1979, Carter continued this transfer process when he outlined military spending projections of over $1 trillion for the coming five-year period (fiscal years 1981 through 1985). In a speech to the National Business Council (an organization composed of the top one-hundred industrialists and bankers), he promised to increase overall military spending each year by at least 5.4 percent

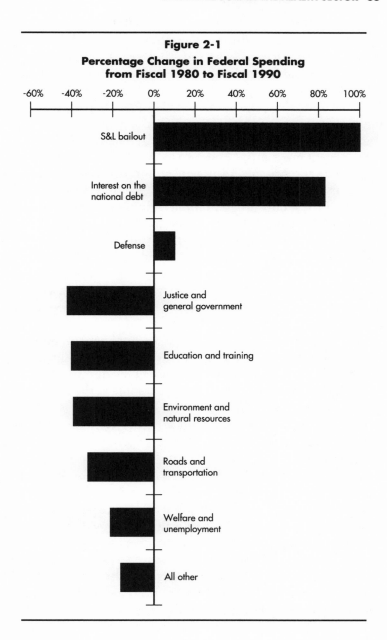

Figure 2-1
**Percentage Change in Federal Spending
from Fiscal 1980 to Fiscal 1990**

more than the rate of inflation.[4] Thus Ronald Reagan did not start the shift of resources—Carter did—but Reagan strengthened a trend Carter had begun by increasing military expenditures by 7.5 percent a year.

At the same time, there was a reduction of 32 percent in the funding for water and navigation projects, 35 percent for mass transit, 70 percent for sewage treatment, 38 percent for low-income benefit programs, 22 percent for Medicaid, 12 percent for basic medical research, and 18 percent for federal public health programs. The list could go on and on. As the 1986 Economic Report of the Council of Economic Advisors to the President reported: "The reduction in domestic outlays financed by general revenues [was] thus slightly more than sufficient to balance the increase in defense spending and interest costs.... One implication of the very substantial reduction in non-defense spending [was] that it permit[ted] an increase in defense spending without an equal increase in tax revenue."[5] Figure 2-1 shows these changes.

These federal cuts and the changes in employment, plus the reduction in employee health benefits described in Chapter 1, were largely responsible for the increase in the number of uninsured during those years, as well as the decline in the utilization of health services (see Table 2-1).

Why did these transfers of funds occur? Why did military expenditures grow so rapidly and social expenditures decline so substantially?

Four major explanations have been put forward by the establishment institutions—the corporate controlled media, the major foundations, and the major academic centers—that set "conventional wisdom." The first is that the growth in military expenditures was essential to "national security," while cuts in social (including health) expenditures were part of the government's response to an anti-government mood that was assumed to prevail. In other words, it was argued that these policies were supported by a "popular mandate."

Table 2-1

Changes in the Number of Insured and the Utilization of Physicians and Hospitals in the United States, 1982–1986

	1982	1986
Percentage of population uninsured	14.0	17.0
Mean number of physician's visits per person per year		
Insured	3.8	3.2
Uninsured	4.7	4.4
Percentage hospitalized		
Insured	5.2	4.6
Uninsured	8.5	5.7
Percentage without a physician's visit in the past year	19.0	33.0
Percentage without a usual source of care	11.0	18.0

The second explanation is that federal social (including health) expenditures had grown so large that they were contributing to the economic recession. This assumed that these expenditures were partially financed by credit, which was contributing to the federal deficit, perceived to be one of the major causes of our economic difficulties. Thus those expenditures had to be reduced.

The third explanation is that during the 1960s and 1970s government regulation of the workplace (to assure the health and safety of the workers and the environment) interfered with management prerogatives, forcing higher management costs, thus making these enterprises less competitive and contributing to the slowing down of the economy.

And the fourth and final explanation is that the "market" is more efficient than the government in regulating the cost and distribution of health resources. This is why the privatization and commodification of medical and health services was a major trademark of all federal policies during these years. Both the executive and legislative branches carried out policies that favored intervention by the private sector to solve our health problems.

These four explanations continue to provide the framework for federal health policy. It is important, therefore, that we analyze them one by one to see what evidence there is to support or refute them. We must always be skeptical of "conventional wisdom" and look at the facts behind it.

THE OFFICIAL RATIONALE FOR THE AUSTERITY POLICIES OF THE 1980S

Was There a Popular Mandate for the Austerity Policies of the 1980s?

In a country that claims to be a democracy, the argument that the austerity policies of the past thirteen years were carried out in response to a popular mandate carries enormous weight. It legitimizes those policies. In this respect, the elections of Ronald Reagan and George Bush were interpreted by both conservatives and liberals as reflecting a popular wish to reduce the size and role of government—except in the military area. Just a few months after the 1980 election, Congress passed legislation that substantially reduced the level of social (including health) spending. Senator Daniel Patrick Moynihan told his colleagues on the Budget Committee that by responding to the "popular mood and mandate, we have undone thirty years of social legislation in three days."[6] The vote was unanimous, and included such leading liberals as Gary Hart of Colorado, Howard M. Metzenbaum of Ohio, and Donald W. Riegle, Jr. of Michigan.

In the health sector, David Rogers and Robert Blendon, then president and vice-president of the Robert Wood Johnson Foundation, the largest and most influential health services research foundation in the country, wrote in the *New England Journal of Medicine* that government health expenditures had to be cut following the popular mandate expressed in the electoral process.

In all of these explanations, "popular mandate" becomes the motor behind health policies that, as I will show later, had a very

Table 2-2

**Percentage Who Want a Tax-Financed
National Health Plan**

Date	Poll	Percent Support
1989	NBC (national)	67
1989	Louisville Courier Journal (Kentucky)	62
1990	Los Angeles Times (national)	72
1990	Atlantic Financial (West Virginia)	62
1990	CBS/New York Times (national)	64
1990	Gallup for Blue Cross (national)	60
1990	Hartford Courant (Connecticut)	60
1990	Roper (national)	69
1990	Associated Press (national)	62

negative impact on the health and well-being of the population. This supposed anti-government mood was also used to explain President Clinton's recent move to cut the size of the federal government by 100,000 jobs. It is important, therefore, that we look for any evidence that there *was* a popular mandate to carry out those policies. But how do we recognize a popular mandate when we see one? In other words, how do we know what people want? One way is to analyze people's responses to opinion polls; another is to analyze election results.

Although we must be cautious in interpreting polls because people's responses depend on how the questions are phrased and how the polls are administered, they can still help us understand what people want. In the case of the government's role in health care, the evidence is overwhelming: poll after poll has shown that the vast majority wants an *expansion* of government health expenditures and *strengthening* of government regulations that protect workers, consumers, and the environment. In fact, as Table 2-2 shows, the majority wants a government-financed and

Figure 2-2
Satisfaction with Health Care, by Nation, in 1990

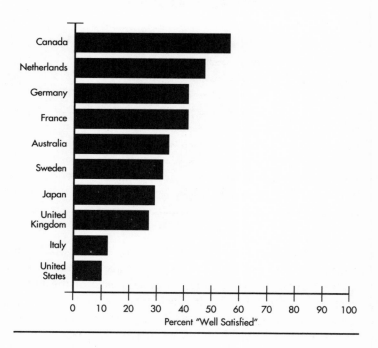

Percent "Well Satisfied"

administered national health program that is comprehensive and covers everyone.

Further, as Figure 2-2 shows, in no other country are people as dissatisfied with their health care as they are in the United States. People's support for such a program increases as their income declines. According to the polls, then, there is *no* mandate to carry out the policies being followed by the government.

How is it that people elected presidents in 1980, 1984, and 1988 who were so committed to policies opposed by the majority of the population? To answer this question, we need to turn our

Table 2-3

**Percentage of Electorate That Voted
for Presidential Candidates**

	1976	1980	1984	1988	1992
Republican	26	27	32	28	21
Democrat	27	22	21	23	28
Independent	0	3	0	0	7
Total	53	52	53	51	56

attention to Table 2-3, which shows the percentage of the electorate that voted for Ford, Carter, Reagan, Bush, and Clinton.

From this table we can draw several conclusions. The first is
that the majority of the population did not vote for these presidents. Another, and equally important, point is that almost half
of the population did not vote *at all*. Since there is a direct
relationship between income and electoral participation (the
higher the income, the more likely a person is to vote, and vice
versa), we can conclude that the majority of the *working class* did
not vote. Remember that this is the class that most strongly
supports the establishment of a national health program and is
most aware that the government does not represent its interests.

Based on these facts, it is hard to see how anyone can say that
there has been a "popular mandate" to reduce the size and role
of government in the health sector. And that argument is even
more difficult to sustain when we learn that even those who did
vote for Reagan and Bush in 1980, 1984, and 1988, often indicated
in exit polls that they disagreed with the health policies of both.
They wanted a larger, rather than a smaller, role for government
in the health sector. And in the 1992 election, the second most
important issue for Clinton's supporters, after job security, was
his promise to provide a national health program. Thus we can
conclude that there has been a popular mandate during the 1980s

and 1990s to do precisely the *opposite* of what the government has been doing.

Is The Government's Role in the Health Sector Too Great and Is this Contributing to the Economic Crisis?

One of the four explanations for our economic difficulties is that the level of government expenditure on health is too high and that this is contributing to the federal budget deficit. But in fact government spending on the health sector is rather meager. Compared to the governments of other capitalist countries, the U.S. government allocates less to health care and provides fewer benefits in those programs it does provide. In Sweden, government expenditures make up 91.7 percent of all health care expenditures and in Germany they make up 77.1 percent—compared to only 41.7 percent in the United States. Put another way, in Sweden 8.2 percent of the GNP goes to public expenditures on health, in Germany 7.8 percent, and in the United States only 4.7 percent. The U.S. government spends too little rather than too much on health care. Further, all the countries with larger government health expenditures have better economic indicators than the United States—less unemployment, lower rates of inflation, and higher rates of economic growth. Thus the meager amounts the U.S. government spends on health care cannot be considered responsible for our economic problems.

The United States also provides less comprehensive benefits than most countries at a similar level of economic development. The majority of U.S. citizens are not covered by any government program, and the programs that do exist—such as Medicaid, which covers only 40 percent of the medically indigent, and Medicare, which covers only 52 percent of all expenditures made by the elderly—are far from comprehensive. The majority of the elderly in the other advanced capitalist countries have some form of government help to pay for pharmaceuticals, for example, help that does not exist under Medicare.

Are U.S. Government Regulations Too Protective of Workers, Consumers, and the Environment? Are the Social Costs of That Protection Responsible for the Uncompetitiveness of the Economy?

The best way to respond to these questions is to share with you an experience I had at an international conference on occupational health policy held in Bologna, Italy, in the fall of 1992. The conference was sponsored by the major European trade unions and was attended by trade union representatives from all over the world, including the United States. The United States was represented by a trade unionist from California named Helena Martínez. She remained silent during most of the conference, while her brothers and sisters from other advanced capitalist nations discussed the state of the occupational health services and the rights of workers in their own countries. At the very end, she stood up and gave one of the most moving speeches of the conference. I wish it could have been on prime-time TV in the United States. It was an angry talk. She told the conference that what she had heard had had a dramatic effect on her life. She had always been told that U.S. workers are better off than workers in other countries, and she had believed it. But in listening to her brothers and sisters at the conference, she had come to realize how little she and her fellow workers had in comparison with Italian, French, German, Scandinavian, Spanish, and other European workers. She went on to denounce the misinformation that makes working Americans believe that they have it best, a belief so widespread that working people have been blinded to the poverty of their rights: "We do not have it better; we have it worse than the majority of workers in other countries like ours. Why was I not told about this reality which I have discovered in this conference?"

Helena Martínez was absolutely right, of course. U.S. workers have less, not more, government protection than workers in other developed countries. You can see the dramatic difference by comparing—to use only one example—the health rights guar-

Table 2-4
Rights of Safety Delegates and Safety Committees in Sweden and the United States

Right	Sweden	United States
Right to be consulted prior to changes in the work process	+	−
Right to bring in consultant paid by management	+	−
Right to mandatory health and safety training for all new workers	+	−
Right to be trained for monitoring	+	−
Hiring and firing of occupational physicians and engineers	+	−
Right of workers' safety delegates to stop work	+	−
Right of inspectors to stop work	+	−

anteed by national legislation to the majority of workers in Sweden with the rights guaranteed by national legislation or collective bargaining agreements in the United States (Table 2-4). In Sweden, workers have a voice in the hiring and firing of occupational health professionals. It is unthinkable that the workers at Bethlehem Steel could hire and fire their occupational health doctors. These doctors are hired and fired by management, and are accountable only to management. The United States protects the health and safety of workers much less than do the governments of other advanced capitalist countries.

A similar situation exists with regard to environmental protection. As Table 2-5 shows, environmental conditions during the 1970s and 1980s, when the corporate class was complaining that the government was going too far in protecting the environment, were worse than in other advanced capitalist countries, including those with better economic performances. Government regula-

Table 2-5
Pollution Levels in Selected Countries in 1975

Country	Carbon Monoxide	Hydrocarbons	Nitrogen Oxides
	Emissions per capita (kg)		
United States	402	122	103
Sweden	171	52	38
West Germany	—	30	31
Japan	—	—	20
Austria	129	6	15
	Emissions per unit of energy consumed (tons/103 tons of energy)		
United States	51	69	13
Sweden	29	15	6
West Germany	—	8	8
Japan	—	—	7
Austria	42	2	3

tion to protect the environment is for the most part weaker in the United States. As one Senate report put it, the available evidence "does not convict U.S. regulations of decreasing competitiveness with other nations. The United States, for example, has less stringent air quality objectives than a number of major competitors."[7]

Not only are the environmental regulations weaker in the United States, but industry's investment in environmental controls is lower than in other advanced capitalist countries. The truth of this struck me a few years ago when several public health professionals in Baltimore, where I live, tried to impress on the people who run Bethlehem Steel's Baltimore operations the need to reduce the amount of pollution generated by its mills. (Visitors to Baltimore may notice that when they walk in the lovely Harborplace, there is often a spectacular reddish sunset on the southeast horizon. This is the result of the enormous pollution coming from the steel mills.) Bethlehem Steel resisted the call for a larger investment in pollution controls, arguing that it could not afford the cost and remain competitive with the Japanese. The company then pressured the government to reduce even further the limited federal funds allocated to protecting the environment. For instance, between 1971 and 1977, when the steel giants were asking that federal regulations be weakened, these same corporations were investing considerably less in pollution controls than was the Japanese steel industry. In no way can such limited investment in environmental protection be considered responsible for the problems faced by the steel industry—or by any other industry, for that matter.

Is Market Intervention More Efficient Than Government Intervention in Regulating the Cost and Distribution of Health Resources?

The United States is the only advanced capitalist country in which both the majority of funds for the health sector (58 percent) and the overwhelming majority of providers—physicians, hospitals, nursing homes, and others—are private. If the market-oriented private sector was more efficient than the public sector in controlling costs and distributing health resources to the majority of the population, then we would expect the entire health care sector to have lower costs per capita and to provide better benefits than other countries where the funding is public. The reality, however, is exactly the opposite. Figure 2-3 shows how the United States spends more than any other country on health care per capita. Yet people in the United States have more limited benefits. In other countries, doctors' bills, hospital fees, lab costs, convalescent and nursing home care, drugs and medicines, eyeglasses, and ordinary dental care are all covered, in whole or in part, for the entire population. In the United States, they are only covered for the poor and aged—and then not always in full.

The United States also has the most administrative waste:

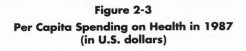

Figure 2-3
Per Capita Spending on Health in 1987
(in U.S. dollars)

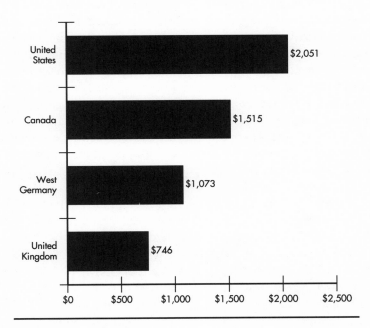

nearly 25 percent of all health expenditures go to paper shuffling. It is difficult, in the light of these facts, to conclude that the private sector is better able than the public sector to control costs or provide coverage.

THE REAL REASON FOR THE AUSTERITY POLICIES

Having analyzed the establishment's explanations for the austerity policies of the last thirteen years and shown them to be wrong, let us look at an alternative answer to the extremely important question of why there has been such a large increase in military expenditures and such a dramatic decline in social expenditures.

These trends are related: they are two sides of the same coin. The reactionary sector of the corporate class has had very close connections with the military establishment, responsible for national security. These connections led to what President Eisenhower called the military-industrial complex, and this complex wields enormous power. The military budget is vital to the interests of many of the most powerful voices of the corporate class. Sixty-five of the top one-hundred corporations are significantly involved in military contracts. But military contracts are just the tip of the iceberg. There are indirect subcontractors, producers of intermediary goods and parts, and suppliers of raw materials, all of which place military spending at the very heart of the economy.

Actually, to fully measure the impact of military expenditures on the economy, we must consider not only the direct expenses that go into producing military hardware, but the additional consumer goods purchased by those who receive military dollars. Direct military expenditures (13 percent of GNP),[8] plus indirect consumer expenditures (12 to 13 percent of GNP), add up to 25 or 26 percent of GNP. The military-industrial complex is characterized by (1) very high profits, the second largest after the pharmaceutical industry; (2) a very stable source of capital through government contracts; (3) the absence of specific interest groups that could develop private alternatives—there are no private armies to compete with the armed forces; (4) a monopoly in the selling of services; and (5) a clear linkage during the last thirteen years between military-corporate industry and branches of government, such as the top echelons of the Department of Defense and the congressional committees that are supposed to oversee defense spending.

The primary source of capital for the military industry is tax money—that is, public money. This money is diverted from health and social expenditures. It is not by chance that the major voices in Congress, industry, and academia that were calling for higher military expenditures were the same voices that supported cuts in social (including health) expenditures. The transfer from the social to the military sectors has had a devastating effect on the well-being of the population. Cities whose coffers were almost empty sent enough dollars to the Pentagon in one week to cover their entire deficits. The growth of military expenditure was therefore based in part on the impoverishment of the quality of life—responsible, in part, for the 40 percent increase in the number of robberies on our streets, where, on average, an American has a higher probability of being murdered than an American soldier had of being killed during World War II; where 85 percent of the elderly are afraid to walk more than half a mile away from home; where a handgun is sold every 13 seconds and a child is murdered every three hours; and where a child dies of poverty every 53 minutes. All of this occurs in this rich land of ours, with a government committed to national "security."

During the past thirteen years, we have also seen a decline in the percentage of the population covered by health services, an increase in the number of people who did not receive any health care at all, a decline in the number of physician's visits, and increases in the percentage of out-of-pocket expenses paid by working people (and the elderly), including copayments and deductibles.

This reduction in social expenditures was a reaction to the achievements of the previous two decades. During the 1960s and early 1970s there was an *increase* in social expenditures and an *expansion* of government regulations to protect workers, consumers, and the environment. During these same decades, there was an average of one revolution per year somewhere in the world. These achievements posed a clear threat to the interests of corporate America, which responded by aggressively attacking the standard of living of the working population in order to weaken and divide it, to lower its level of expectation. The reductions in entitlements and social services in the 1980s were therefore important elements in a policy that was aimed at weakening the working population. For instance, people who lose their health insurance when they lose their jobs are less willing to stand up to their employers than they might be if they received health coverage regardless of where (or whether) they were employed. Also, the heightening of racism and sexism was aimed at dividing rather than uniting the working population.

Here it is important to stress two points. The first concerns the ways in which a health program can divide rather than unite people. If, for example, you were to ask white steelworkers whether they are willing to pay higher taxes for a health program that will benefit black children whose parents are unemployed, they will probably say no. You may feel that such a response is motivated by racism, and although I cannot exclude that possibility, the real explanation is probably much more complex. The steelworker's family is under enormous stress. Its disposable income (the money it has available to spend) has been reduced since 1972, even though more family members are working. Its health benefits have also been reduced, while copayments and deductibles have increased. How can the white steelworker endorse a tax increase that will benefit someone else?

If, however, the same steelworkers are asked whether they are willing to pay higher taxes for a national health program that will benefit *all* children—their own as well as the children of the unemployed—they will answer yes. Solidarity is always a better motivation than compassion. Universal programs unite people; programs that provide different levels of benefits to different people depending on their means divide people.

The reactionary policies of the 1980s, initiated in the late 1970s and continued into the early 1990s, had been thoroughly discredited by 1992. The election of Bill Clinton was an indicator of that. People are desperate for change. Will they get it? We turn now to an examination of the prospects for change under the Democratic Party.

3

THE DEMOCRATIC PARTY AND THE FUTURE OF HEALTH CARE IN THE UNITED STATES

By the end of the thirteen years described in the previous chapter, the situation in the health care sector had deteriorated dramatically. The proportion of the population not covered by insurance had increased by 22 percent, the amount of direct out-of-pocket expenses had increased by 42 percent, the mode of funding health services became even more regressive, and the funds going into administration quadrupled. While the costs of health care increased and health benefits declined for most people, the profits of the health insurance and pharmaceutical industries, and the incomes of physicians, increased. Average earnings for doctors climbed from $89,900 in 1981 to $164,300 in 1992—

well above either inflation or the increase in income of the average family. The top twenty drug companies saw their profits increased 15 percent per year over the past ten years (compared with an average annual increase of 3.2 percent for the top Fortune 500 companies). The compensation of top executives of the twenty-six most important health care corporations, which was already fifty-four times the salary of a nurse in 1985, increased to eighty-five times that salary in 1992. And hospital profits increased by 23 percent in the year 1992 alone. Today, the highest paid person in the United States is Thomas F. Frist, Jr., the chief executive officer of Hospital Corporation of America, who makes $127 million a year!

The top people were doing very well indeed. The majority, however, were not. Their health care situation was deteriorating: they had to pay more but received less care. Not surprisingly, they were fed up and wanted a major change. According to a Harris poll taken on January 5, 1993, 49 percent of Americans felt that "the American health care system has so much wrong that it needs to be completely rebuilt," while another 32 percent wanted to see profound changes in the health care sector.[1]

What are the major characteristics of this system at this point in time? Here it is useful to review some of the data supplied in Chapter 1:

(1) *It is not universal.* Seventeen percent of all Americans, 28 percent of African-Americans, and 32 percent of Hispanics do not have any form of health insurance.

(2) *It is not comprehensive.* Americans spend more in out-of-pocket expenses than the citizens of any other advanced capitalist country (see Figure 3-1). Moreover, the overwhelming majority do not have coverage for long-term care.

(3) *It is not secure.* Sixty-two percent of working people—those whose employers self-insure their employees—can have their health insurance dropped if their condition requires treatment that is considered too expensive.

(4) *It is not fair.* The head of General Motors, who makes $1.8

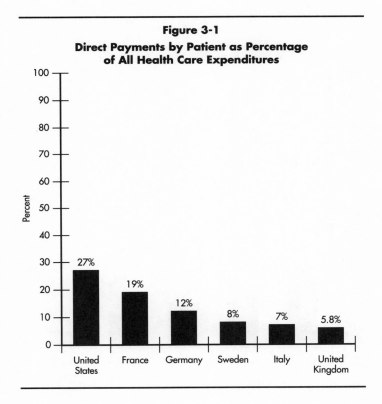

Figure 3-1

**Direct Payments by Patient as Percentage
of All Health Care Expenditures**

million a year, pays the same premium for his health care as an unskilled assembly line worker in a General Motors plant.

(5) *It is inefficient.* Twenty-five cents out of every health dollar are spent on administration and paper shuffling. As Figure 3-2 shows, no other country spends this much on the administration of its health services.

Not surprisingly, the level of discontent with the financing and organization of health care has reached an all-time high. People are angry; they want change. This mood was responsible for the victory of a virtually unknown candidate in the 1992 race for the Senate in Pennsylvania. Senator Harris Wofford, who made

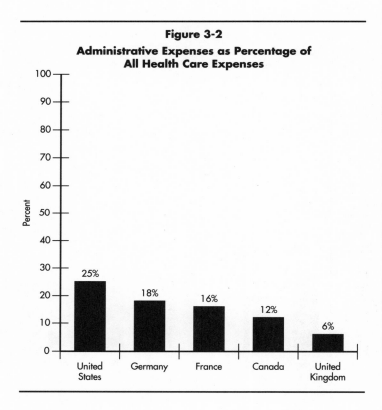

Figure 3-2
**Administrative Expenses as Percentage of
All Health Care Expenses**

health care reform the major item in his platform, defeated Richard Thornburgh, the favored establishment candidate and a friend of George Bush. And everywhere else, poll after poll showed that health care reform was the second most important issue in the campaign. The same polls showed that the two major concerns about health care were its *cost,* with nearly 50 percent of the population reporting that it was having difficulty paying for health care, and *insecurity,* with 60 percent worried about losing its coverage. The growing privileges for the few—the profits earned by the medical-industrial complex—were based on the growing problems of the many.

Side by side with the desire for change is an equally threatening event for the medical-industrial complex: a growing demand for what has become known as the "single-payer" alternative—a government-funded and administered health service in which the government contracts directly with providers for the delivery of health services, bypassing the insurance companies. A February 1992 Harris poll found that 69 percent of the population wanted a government-funded and government-run health service, with the single-payer model being the preferred choice. The Canadians have such a system. Canadians have a health card that allows them to choose their provider; there are no copayments, no deductibles, and no fee for service.

What is threatening to the U.S. medical-industrial complex is that Canada once had a health care system similar to ours. Canada also had the insurance industry—including the Blues and the commercial insurance companies—running its health sector. In 1972, however, the Canadian parliament passed the National Health Program Act, which nationalized the funding of health care and eliminated the role of the insurance industry. The government now sets the rates for the health care providers, including hospital budgets and physicians' fees. Since the National Health Program was established, Canadians have been able to control costs while expanding—rather than reducing, as in the United States—health benefits (see Figure 3-3).

We can see how this model threatens the medical-industrial complex. Under a single-payer system, some elements of the complex would see their incomes and privileges either considerably reduced or eliminated altogether. Physicians, for instance, earn 25 percent less in Canada than in the United States, while pharmaceutical prices are 30 percent lower. The health insurance industry would be completely eliminated. The insurance industry is fully aware of this. Dr. Carl Schramm, president of the Health Insurance Association of America (HIAA), has defined the current struggle as one of life or death for the insurance industry.

Figure 3-3

**Health Care Costs in the United States and Canada
as Percentage of GNP, 1960–1991**

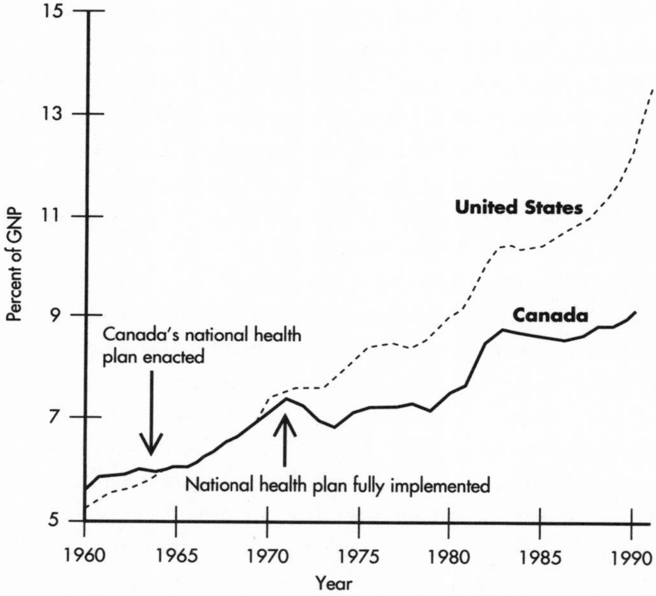

HIAA has spent $20 million on a campaign to defeat the single-payer model.

MANAGED COMPETITION: CORPORATE AMERICA'S RESPONSE TO THE HEALTH CARE CRISIS

The medical-industrial complex has had to respond to the growing unrest. Its response is called "managed competition." This model was first proposed by Alain Enthoven, professor of economics at Stanford University and a member of the Jackson Hole group, an informal group whose members represent the large insurance companies (whose interests conflict with those of the small insurance companies), some of the largest corporate employers, the pharmaceutical industry, and some of the major professional associations. The Jackson Hole group's analysis of the health care crisis is that it is due to a lack of competition in the health sector. According to this theory, Americans are not sufficiently cost conscious when they buy health insurance because it is paid for by their employers. As a result, they are often overinsured and also often overuse health care resources, a tendency that is encouraged by fee-for-service providers (who benefit from this overconsumption). The solution, according to Enthoven and the Jackson Hole group, is for the government to discipline the workers as consumers—by making them more cost conscious—and for the insurance industry to discipline the providers—by making them work in insurance-controlled provider networks or managed-care plans. This disciplining would be done by taxing health benefits over and above a basic or benchmark level. These taxes would mean that consumers would pay more for their health benefits, which would in turn make them more cost conscious and would encourage them to select the cheaper and more cost-effective basic plans.

For their part, the providers would be forced to work in managed-care plans that would be controlled by the large insurance companies. The providers would become employees of, or contract their services with, these insurers, which would force them to practice in a cautious and cost-saving manner. The consumer would be required to enroll in an insurance-controlled managed-care plan—accentuating the trend toward the domination of the health care industry by the large insurance companies that was described in Chapter 1. When this process began over twenty years ago, it was predicted by Paul Ellwood, another major theorist of managed competition, that insurer-controlled HMOs (health maintenance organizations, or prepaid group practices) would "stimulate a course of change in the health industry that would have some of the classical aspects of the industrial revolution—conversion to larger units of production, technological innovation, division of labor, substitution of capital for labor, vigorous competition and profitability as the mandatory condition for survival."[2] Every major insurance company—Metropolitan Life, Aetna, Prudential, Connecticut General, and the Blues, among others—either has managed-care plans, is acquiring existing ones, or is developing new ones of its own. Insurer-controlled HMOs will be corporate assembly-line capitalism for the majority, while the elites will continue to enjoy free choice and fee-for-service medical care. As Alain Enthoven and Richard Kronick have written, "What about traditional fee per services individual and single speciality group practices? We doubt that they would generally be compatible with economic efficiency.... Some would survive in private solo practice without health plan contracts, serving the well-to-do."[3]

According to managed-competition theorists, the competition among insurance-controlled managed-care plans would lead to a decline in the cost of premiums. Insurance-controlled plans would compete among themselves for the premiums paid by employers—who would, of course, choose the least expensive plans for their employees.

The proponents of managed competition are aware of the problems faced by the 38 million Americans who do not have any health benefits. Most of the uninsured are low-wage employees working for small businesses for which the premiums represent a considerable cost. Small employers have to pay much higher premiums because their administrative costs are higher, as Figure 3-4 shows. The managed-competition solution to this problem is to encourage small employers to become part of larger health insurance purchasing cooperatives that would pool the employees of many small enterprises and buy insurance premiums on behalf of their employers. In other words, these cooperatives would act as the purchasing agents for the small employers, as well as for individuals who could not afford to buy health insurance on the open market.

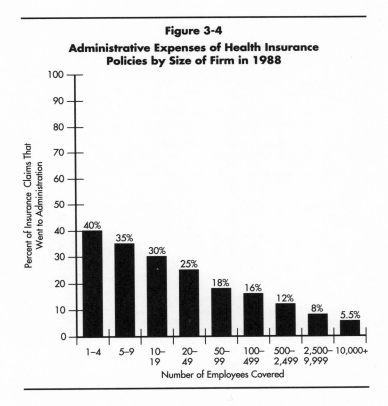

Figure 3-4

Administrative Expenses of Health Insurance Policies by Size of Firm in 1988

WHAT'S WRONG WITH MANAGED COMPETITION?

It is important to grasp that both the understanding of the problem and the solutions put forward by the proponents of managed competition are profoundly faulty. There is abundant evidence to invalidate the basic assumptions behind the managed-competition model. The first is that people are not cost conscious and that this is because they do not pay enough of their own health care costs. Figure 3-1 showed how people in the United States pay more in out-of-pocket expenses than do people in any other advanced capitalist society. Americans are well aware of this: the most frequent complaint about health care is its high

Table 3-1
Americans Rank Their Health Care Concerns

Percent worrying "A great deal"/ "Quite a lot . . ."	Total
. . . that health insurance will become so expensive that I won't be able to afford it.	61
. . . that I will have to pay very expensive medical bills not covered by health insurance.	50
. . . that I will not be able to get the health care I need when I am very ill because I can't afford it.	48
. . . that my benefits under my current health care plan will be cut back substantially.	48
. . . that if I have large medical bills, my health plan will refuse to insure me.	39
. . . that my employer's health care costs will limit my wage increases.	31
. . . that my employer will stop providing me with any health insurance.	26
Compared with other major concerns:	
. . . that I will not be able to maintain my standard of living.	50
. . . that I or my spouse will lose our jobs in 1992.	33

cost (see Table 3-1). It is ludicrous to accuse the victims—the patients—for problems that are not of their own making.

A second error in the managed-competition argument is the assertion that insurance companies are the best instruments to control both costs and the quality of care. The empirical evidence proves this wrong. Eighty-two percent of the health care delivery system is *already* under some form of managed care that is contracted by, controlled by, and/or influenced by the insurance companies—through HMOs, preferred provider organizations (PPOs), and other forms of prepaid group practice—and their success at controlling costs has been abysmal. Costs in these managed-care systems have grown from 16 percent to 20 percent per year, *more than twice* the annual rate of inflation during the last thirteen years.

The failure to control costs (while raising profits) has been accompanied by an equally abysmal failure to improve the quality of care. In fact, the intervention of the insurance industry in the medical care sector is one of the major reasons for the deterioration in quality. In order to reduce costs, insurers micro-manage the physician-patient relationship in a way that diminishes and impoverishes it. As noted in Chapter 1, major interventions or tests prescribed or advised by a doctor must be approved by the insurance company, whose primary concern is cost. Fifty-four percent of these requests are rejected by insurance-company clerks, who have no medical training. Further, the amount of administration is enormous. One insurance company—Blue Cross—has more administrative employees in the single state of Massachusetts than does the National Health Program in *all* of Canada.

Despite the lack of merit of managed competition, the corporate class and the medical-industrial complex want to sell it to the public as the solution to the medical care crisis. The *New York Times* has published nine editorials and sixty-two articles in support of managed competition. That same paper—whose motto is, "All the News That's Fit to Print"—did not find it fit to print the news that on April 1, 1993, President Clinton was presented with a petition in favor of a single-payer model that had 1 million signatures. In fact, not *one* of the major media reported this event. Four of the twelve members of the *New York Times* board of directors are also on the boards of health-insurance companies.[4]

After Clinton's electoral victory, due in large part to his campaign promise to provide universal and comprehensive health benefits, he appointed a Task Force on National Health Care Reform, headed by his wife Hillary Rodham Clinton. Its initial mandate was to implement a managed-competition plan, as proposed by the Jackson Hole group. Popular pressure for establishing a government-funded and administered national health program has been the major obstacle to the implementation of this plan.

As I write this, the nation is engaged in a major struggle over what health care reform we are going to have. Although this struggle is over health care, it is really a struggle over class power. It is revealing that Enthoven derides the democratic potential of our institutions when he writes: "The U.S. political system is incapable of forcing changes in such powerful constituencies as the insurance industry, the hospital industry, organized medicine, the medical devices industry and the pharmaceutical industry."[5] Enthoven seems to believe that U.S. democracy is a class dictatorship, in which one class—a sector of the corporate class—has overwhelming political influence, tantamount to actual control over the political institutions. But I have lived under a dictatorship—I spent my early youth fighting Franco's dictatorship in Spain. I know how to recognize a dictatorship when I see one, and the United States is not a dictatorship. On the other hand, it is not a fully representative democracy either. People's voices are heard, but they must compete with other, far more influential, voices that define what is or is not possible in the realm of change. Change can occur. But it will require an enormous mobilization around a progressive health care reform in which the majority of the population, rather than a minority, will control their health care institutions. Is this mobilization possible in the United States? To answer this question we need to understand how health care reforms have occurred in other developed capitalist countries. This is the topic of the next chapter.

4

CLASS POWER AND HEALTH CARE: WHY THE UNITED STATES IS DIFFERENT

The U.S. population has wanted a humane and comprehensive national health program for a long time, but has not gotten it. Why? In Chapter 1 we saw that the answer to this question lies in the nature of power, and in particular class power, in our society. As we shall see in what follows, it is the nature of class relations in any society that is the primary determinant of its type of health services. We therefore need to understand the class structure of these societies: the classes, their political and economic institutions (unions, political parties, chambers of commerce, etc.) and their influence on the policymaking bodies and, in particular, on the state. We need to understand not only the power now held by these class forces, but the power they had in the past. Indeed, our present is the realization of our past.

Two classes have historically played major roles in shaping a country's health services: the capitalist class and the working class. How these two classes are related to each other and to other classes is critical to understanding the type of funding and organization of the health services. The capitalist class and the working class have historically had different and even opposite views on how to structure health care. The United States provides a clear example of this.

THE LABOR MOVEMENT AND ITS POSITION ON HEALTH CARE

In the nineteenth century, working-class organizations developed friendly societies and voluntary sickness funds to assure the continuation of income and the provision of medical care when workers and their families were sick. As their name indicates, the sickness funds were voluntary and were controlled by fraternal orders (such as, in the United States, the Knights of Labor). The fraternities, which were the predecessors of today's trade unions, used these funds as a way of attracting new members to the labor movement.

In the United States, the labor movement was the first force to demand that the state play a role in providing health care. The American Federation of Labor (AFL), which organized the craft unions (such as the cigarmakers, iron workers, and carpenters), at first preferred an employer-based insurance plan, but this preference lasted only until Samuel Gompers, the AFL's first president, retired in 1924. The more militant Congress of Industrial Organizations (CIO), which led the drive to unionize on an industry-wide basis (in such industries as auto, electrical, steel, and rubber), supported universal health benefits from the beginning. After the AFL and CIO merged in 1955, the union movement advocated, at least in theory, universal health benefits for

Table 4-1

Selected Welfare State Characteristics in Scandinavia, Austria, and Germany During the Postwar Period: Means-tested Social (Including Health) Expenditures as a Percentage of Total Social Security Expenditures

Years	Denmark	Norway	Sweden	Austria	Germany
1950	13.2	11.0	11.8	10.1	15.4
1974–1975	1.0	2.1	1.0	2.8	4.9

workers and their families. In doing so, the AFL-CIO joined with the labor movement in all the other advanced capitalist countries.

The major health policy demands of the labor movement in all developed capitalist countries have been: (1) universal health benefits, (2) control by and/or participation of the labor movement in directing the health care system, (3) government responsibility for the management of the funds, and (4) the funding of health care through a system of progressive taxation. These demands have been part of larger demands that would separate the right to benefits from employment, institutionalize state responsibility for universal programs that benefit everyone, and redistribute income and resources from the capitalist class to the working class.[1]

The principle of universality was of paramount importance to the working class because it fostered the key principle of the labor movement—class solidarity—over class fragmentation. Thus from the very beginning the labor movement was against health care benefits being tied to either wages or economic sector. It was also against means-testing as a method of determining the right to benefits.[2] In the Scandinavian countries, in Germany, and in Austria, when socialist parties (meaning social democratic, socialist, or labor parties) came to power, one of their first acts was to eliminate and/or reduce means-tested programs (see Table 4-1).[3]

As part of the struggle for universality, the labor movement fought for uniform levels of benefits, as well as for the coordination or integration of the different publicly administered or licensed insurance funds that provided benefits for different sectors of the working population. And as part of the process of divorcing health benefits from employment, the labor movement fought to shift their funding from payroll taxes to taxes on general revenue, in turn based on progressive taxation.

The capitalist class opposed each of these demands. By favoring the granting of different levels of benefits to different types of workers and the use of means-tests, the capitalist class sought to break working-class solidarity. Private health insurance tied to the job strengthens the employees' attachment to work and the employer, and also increases inequalities among workers, favoring the strongest over the weakest. As Gosta Esping-Andersen has written, "By explicitly targeting legislation to workers and by promoting sharp status distinctions, the political aim was to build and consolidate status cleavages among the wage-earner population. The strategy, in other words, was to thwart broader class formation."[4]

CLASS POWER AS AN EXPLANATION OF NATIONAL HEALTH POLICY

The extent to which either the capitalist class or the working class has been able to reach its objectives in any particular country has depended on the power of each class to influence public policy. For the working class, its power has depended on the following six conditions: (1) The *degree of unionization* of the labor force: the higher the level of unionization, the stronger the labor movement. (2) The *type of union organization*: industrial unionism (which organizes by industry, such as the automobile, steel, or electrical industries) provides more class power than craft unionism (which organizes by trade, such as carpenters, iron workers, or brick layers). Similarly, close coordination within a strong central union federation, which bargains for the entire labor force, allows for labor to make more demands than does a highly decentralized sectoral bargaining process. (3) The *unity* of the labor movement: a movement that is not divided into confessional (e.g., Christian and lay) or political (e.g., socialist, social democratic, or communist) unions is stronger than one that is divided. (4) A *close link* between the labor movement and a political party that represents the interests of the working class and allied popular forces. (5) The *absence of major political divisions* within the working class. (6) A strong *working-class party* that has held power, either alone or in a coalition with other parties.[5]

These six conditions determine the ability of the working-class instruments—political parties and trade unions—to attain their demands. Power, however, is relative: by this I mean that the power of the working class also depends on two other conditions: (1) The ability of this class to establish alliances with other classes, such as farmers and the middle strata of technical-professional workers. For example, in Sweden the early commitment to a comprehensive and universal health program (as well as to other components of the welfare state) was possible primarily because of the alliance between the working-class Social Democratic Party and the Farmers' Party.[6] No such alliance was forged in France and Italy, which explains why similar programs in those countries did not develop until much later. Similarly, the highly popular New Deal programs in the United States in the 1930s (which formed the basis of the U.S. welfare state) were primarily the outcome of an alliance between the working class of the northeastern urban centers and southern farmers.[7] (2) The power and unity (or disunity) of the capitalist class. When the capitalist class is divided among different parties, as in Sweden, the ability of a united working-class party to stimulate change is greater than when the capitalist class is united in a single major party, as in Austria and Italy.

How does this help explain why some countries have a national

Table 4-2
Timing of Establishment of Working-Class Socialist Parties, Major Trade Union Federations, and First Social (including Health) Insurance Schemes

	Socialist Party	Trade Union	Social Insurance
Germany	1875	1868	1883
Austria	1888–89	1893	1888
Denmark	1878	1898	1891
Norway	1887	1877	1894
France	1905	1895	1898
Belgium	1889	1910	1900
Netherlands	1894	1905	1901
Britain	1900	1868	1908
Switzerland	1888	1880	1911
Sweden	1889	1898	1913
Italy	1892	1906	1914

health service, some have national health insurance, and the United States does not have either? First, the establishment of a national health program is related to the strength of the labor movement, realized through its unions and political parties. Second, the different types of funding and organization of the health services are also related to the degree to which the differing class aims in the health sector have been achieved, which in turn depends on the relative power of the two classes.

Table 4-2 shows a clear correlation among the times when a major working-class party was organized, the time a major trade union federation was organized, and the time when the first social insurance (including health insurance) program was established.[8]

Many people associate the development of social insurance programs with the process of industrialization. In this scenario, industrialization created insecurity and social security programs were set up to resolve it. But if this were the case, Belgium and Great Britain, the first two countries to become industrialized, would have been the first to have social security programs. They were not. The reason is that in these countries the working class did not develop its own political party until later. The craft nature of the unions in both countries helps explain the rather late development of such a party.

In summary, then, the critical force behind the birth of health and other social insurance programs was the political and economic strength of the working class. The presence or absence of a national health program in any one country depends on the correlation of forces in that country. The evolution of the different types of funding and organization of health services—in particular, what we can call the "corporate" and "liberal" models—also depended on the alignment of class forces.

The Corporate Health Care Model

The corporate model developed in Germany, Austria, France, and Italy, countries where the new capitalist class was weak, unable to break with the feudal order, and thus had to ally with the feudal aristocracies against the growing strength of the working class. In these states, policies were aimed at (1) dividing the working class by creating differences in the level of health benefits (by making them dependent on work-related contributions), and (2) directing class loyalties away from the universalist appeals of socialism and toward allegiance to the employer. Social and health policies in these countries were aimed at the privileged sectors of the working class: a range of benefits was established so that those at the bottom—the poor—would be taken care of by charity, under religious auspices, while the best-paid workers would receive the highest level of benefits.

Germany was the first country to develop this model. The conservative forces within the dominant power bloc were threatened by a growing working class, organized in the Social Democratic Party. Pressure from this party was responsible for the establishment of the first Health Security Act, in 1888, although the specific event that led to the act occurred not in Germany but in France. In 1871, the Parisian working class took over Paris and established the first-ever workers' state—called the Paris Commune. This uprising had an enormous impact on Bismarck, the German Chancellor, whose major concern became avoiding a similar occurrence in Germany. Consequently, Germany developed a two-pronged policy: repression of the leadership of the Social Democratic Party accompanied by the establishment of a national health insurance program. The program was administered by different funds that covered different types of workers and provided different levels of benefits. These funds were licensed, supervised, and administered by different branches of the state.

It is important to note that while the threat posed by the working-class political party was the stimulus for the Health Security Act, the way in which the act was developed, organized, and administered was determined by the capitalist class. By providing different levels of benefits according to social status and occupation, and by having the state administer each level, the capitalist class tried to divide the workers and weaken class solidarity.

The legacy of these origins can be seen in the German National Health Insurance System today. Its funding is public (from payroll taxes) but the delivery of health services is private. In addition, it is still divided into different funds: those for white-collar workers are different from those for blue-collar workers, and have different benefits. Moreover, the top 10 percent of the population is outside the system, covered primarily by private insurance companies. The German model has been discussed as a possibility for the United States by some leaders of the Democratic Party and by some white-collar sectors of the labor movement.

The Liberal Model

The liberal model developed in those "New World" societies where the capitalist class did not have to establish alliances with a feudal aristocracy. In these societies, which included the United States, Canada, Australia, and New Zealand, social and health policies much more directly reflect the aims of the capitalist class. In the United States, for instance, health policy has been characterized by (1) a reliance on the market, with its preference for private health insurance, and (2) a strong commitment to means testing as a way to distinguish the "deserving" from the "non-deserving."[9] The reliance on the market emphasizes voluntary membership in insurance plans, with benefits closely tied to employment and with meager public benefits in order to encourage private insurance alternatives.

In such countries, working-class organizations (parties and unions) have traditionally been weak and divided, largely because these are "immigrant" countries in which the working class is divided into ethnic or racial groupings. In the United States, for example, there is no mass-based political party that represents the interests of the working class. Instead, working-class interests have generally been channeled through the Democratic Party, whose leadership has—as we saw in Chapter 1—been dominated by the upper and corporate classes. Nor does the United States have centralized bargaining, with a central labor federation that defends the economic interests of the working class as a whole. Instead, the bargaining process occurs sector by sector—in the automobile or steel industries, for instance.

But the working class in the United States has not been silent. The mobilization of major sectors of the working class, along with its allies in other classes, was the main stimulus for the New Deal, which established such programs as Social Security and unemployment insurance. Social security is not only the most popular welfare program but the most popular social insurance program. Labor also won the passage of the National Labor Relations Act, which for the first time guaranteed workers "the right to self-organization, to form, join, or assist labor organizations, to bargain collectively through representatives of their own choosing, and to engage in concerted activities for the purpose of collective bargaining or other mutual aid or protection."

The capitalist class fought these measures and launched a counterattack, and although the labor movement had never before been so strong, it was not strong enough to force the passage of a national health program. Health benefits continued to be provided and administered primarily by employers, and confined to a small sector of the laboring population.

This limited coverage expanded somewhat during World War II. The war, as noted in Chapter 1, had an enormous impact in the United States. Popular expectations for change soared. Labor was militant. Both the industrial unions of the CIO and the craft unions of the AFL called for a national health program. As the president of the AFL, William Green, put it in 1952, "Facts and logic are on the side of a national health insurance ... sooner or later the program for which labor pleads will be enacted."[10]

The capitalist class continued to oppose labor's demands. Its response, which was on all fronts—ideological, political, and economic—was directed at weakening the working class. Through its enormous influence on Congress, it was able to force the passage of the Taft-Hartley Act in 1947. The act, co-sponsored by Republican Senator Robert Taft and Representative Fred Hartley, banned or circumscribed some of the most important collective bargaining rights gained during the New Deal. After its passage, there was no chance that a national health program would be enacted. Health benefits continue to be covered by collective bargaining agreements that are negotiated industry by industry, agreement by agreement. The result is that 62 percent of working people get their health benefits through their work, which, as we have seen, strengthens inequalities and differentials among wage earners, favoring those sectors that have the strongest muscle at the bargaining table and discriminating against—or even excluding—those that are weakest.[11] This "interest group" behavior—as opposed to class behavior—is encouraged by the law. It undermines class solidarity because sectors of labor that occupy a privileged position are less likely to support public programs that help the less fortunate.

The answer to the question of why we do not have a comprehensive and universal health program is clear: It is because of the weakness of the working class, the absence of a mass-based working-class party, very low levels of unionization, and the strength of the capitalist class. In other "New World" societies, such as Canada, Australia, and New Zealand, mass-based socialist parties have been responsible for establishing national health programs. In the case of Canada, the socialist party was instrumental in establishing a comprehensive and universal health insurance system in the province of Saskatchewan and in later expanding it to the rest of the nation.[12] I will return to this below.

DEVELOPMENTS IN THE HEALTH SECTOR FROM THE 1950S ON

While the basis for the funding and organization of the welfare state (and our health services) was established prior to, during, and immediately after World War II, the real development of the welfare state took place after the war, in the 1950s, 1960s, and 1970s. Measured in terms of both employment and expenditures (whether total expenditures, percentage of overall government expenditures, or percentage of the Gross Domestic Product), public funding for health services grew significantly in all the countries considered so far. Table 4-3 shows this growth in public funding as a percentage of GDP. Sweden, where the working class is strongest, has the highest percentage, while the United States, where the working class is weakest, has the lowest (except for Spain and Portugal).[13]

During this same period, although the forms and organization of funding for health care continued to differ in these countries, some common elements began to appear. For instance, in all but

Table 4-3
Public Funds Spent on Health as Percentage
of GDP, 1960–1983

	1960	1970	1980	1983
Sweden	3.4	6.2	8.8	8.8
United Kingdom	3.4	3.9	5.2	5.5
West Germany	3.2	4.2	6.5	6.6
France	2.5	4.3	6.1	6.6
Italy	3.2	4.8	6.0	6.2
Spain	1.4	2.3	4.3	4.4
Greece	1.7	2.2	3.5	—
Portugal	0.9	1.9	4.2	3.9
Austria	2.9	3.4	4.5	4.6
Australia	2.4	3.2	4.7	4.9
New Zealand	3.3	3.5	4.7	5.3
Canada	2.4	5.1	5.4	6.2
United States	1.3	2.8	4.1	4.5

the United States, universalism became established. In countries with national health insurance plans, health benefits increased and were equalized regardless of wage differentials, while the different public insurance funds were centralized. Even in the United States the population covered by both public and private insurance programs grew, although these programs did not become either universal or comprehensive.

A primary reason for the expansion of health coverage and the move toward universalism was the growing strength of the working class. From the late 1960s into the early 1980s, working-class parties either held power or gained in popularity in many Western capitalist countries. In the mid-1980s, representatives of socialist parties became the largest voting bloc in the European parliament.[14] In the United States, although the labor movement gained strength until the mid-1970s, in part because of the short-age of labor, by the 1980s only 23 percent of the labor force was organized; by 1991, the figure had fallen to 16 percent.

A primary reason for both the expanded coverage and the move toward universalism was the growing strength of the working class. First, the degree of unionization increased in 18 of the top 23 advanced capitalist countries, reaching an all-time high in all but France and the United States in the late 1970s.[15] The great popularity of universal coverage and the existence of socialist parties was a factor even conservatives were forced to deal with. For example, President Reagan was more successful than Prime Minister Thatcher in reducing public expenditures in the health sector not because Americans were less supportive of such expenditures,[16] but because the Conservative Party in Britain had to compete with a working-class Labour Party that was committed to an expansion of health expenditures. In the United States, on the other hand, the Republican Party did not have such competition. On the contrary: the health cuts were carried out with the support of the Democratic Party leadership.

It is important to note that the growing welfare state was characterized by government intervention not only in the realm of distribution, but in the realm of production.[17] In a perceptive analysis of legislative practices in Western Europe, Canadian political scientist Leo Panitch showed how governments were pressured by popular demands to question the sanctity of the private ownership of the means that produced the wealth of these societies. In country after country, governments curtailed employers' prerogatives in the world of production. Governments talked about industrial democracy, economic democracy, worker control, worker co-determination, and other concepts that left employers worried. In Sweden, Great Britain, France, and many other developed countries, socialist demands for changing patterns of class power were enacted. In France, a government was elected on a platform that called for the end of capitalism!

What was true for these economies was also true for their health sectors. In most of these countries, there was an increase in government intervention in the funding and organization of health care. In most, including the United States, government-provided health benefits expanded, while health planning and regulatory programs aimed at guiding and/or directing the reorganization of the health services were established. Occupational health and environmental legislation also grew, with active government intervention that reduced or constrained some of management's prerogatives.

In brief, it was during this period, and particularly in the 1960s and 1970s, that labor strengthened its power, putting the capitalist class on the defensive. This helps explain the strong conservative reaction of the capitalist class when it regained power in the 1980s. Anti-welfare-state policies formed the key elements of conservative austerity measures (as we discussed in Chapter 2). As one of the best-known spokesmen for the "new" British Conservative Party put it, "Old-fashioned Tories say there isn't class war. New Tories make no bones about it; we are class warriors and we expect to be victorious."[18] In a similar fashion, the chairman of Kaiser Aluminum in the United States, Cornell Maier, who was one of the major supporters of the 1980s austerity policies, declared, "This is war. The battle is not over our economic system. The battle is over our political system."[19]

But we cannot conclude from this survey of national health policies that all Western European countries have, by establishing national health programs, evolved toward identical goals. Common elements within these societies—universalism and increasing comprehensiveness—should not be confused with an identity of experience. Far from it. The experiences of the northern European countries have been very different from those of southern Europe. Industrialization took place much earlier in the north than in the south, with the result that the working classes there were better developed and organized politically. The union movements in the north were (and still are) strong and for the most part united. (Between 70 and 80 percent of the labor force in Sweden and Austria is unionized, compared to between 40 and 50 percent in West Germany and Britain and less than 20 percent in France.) Socialist parties were rooted in the labor unions, which were the main force behind them. To use Gramsci's expression, the parties were the "organic instruments" of the unions.

In southern Europe, where industrialization began much later and the working class was (and still is) weaker, a different constellation of class forces developed. On the one hand, the southern European working class has tended to generate more revolutionary traditions than has the working class in the more reformist north—initially anarchists, subsequently communists. But these forces were not the majority within the working class, which therefore remained divided at both the union and political-party levels.[20] On the other hand, the dominant political bloc in southern Europe was, until recently, profoundly conservative, and even on occasion—as in Greece, Spain, and Italy before World War II—fascist. The state was highly centralized and bureaucratic, with a strong military-police apparatus. This had two consequences for national health policy. First, as Table 4-3 showed, public expenditure on health in the post-World War II period was lower in southern than in northern Europe.

Second, the main concern of the southern European socialist parties, once in power, has been to modernize and democratize the state apparatus rather than expand social expenditures. In all these countries, the welfare state remains less developed than in northern Europe.

I want to make it clear that while the working class was the major force behind changes in health policy in the postwar period, it was not the only force: there is no one-to-one correlation between the strength of the working class and these changes. Variations can be attributed to other forces. But the emphasis on class forces is an attempt to remedy the silence on this topic in current explanations of health and social policy. Further, the electoral successes of the working-class parties during the postwar period were largely due to their identification with the interests of the majority of the wage earners, including white-collar employees and the middle strata of technical-professional workers. These alliances have not been easy. For example, these sectors have been willing to join the working class in support of comprehensive and universal health coverage in times of economic security and growth, but in times of austerity these same sectors resented the equalization of benefits and became more receptive to the capitalist-class message that benefits must be linked to wages. These tensions are evident in most developed capitalist countries today.

Finally, an important point worth stressing is that the popular demand for allocating health care resources according to need has always conflicted with the capitalist logic of putting profits first and people's needs second. Every inch of human space in the capitalist order has been won after enormous struggle carried out by working people against the powerful and rich.

WILL THE UNITED STATES HAVE A NATIONAL HEALTH PROGRAM?

As we have seen, the development of the welfare state and one of its main components—a universal and comprehensive government-run health program—is directly related to the strength of the working class and its political and economic instruments. And, as we have noted, the United States is the *only* major capitalist developed country without some form of national health program, and also the only one without a mass-based socialist party (which is in turn largely due to the weakness of its unions). We have to conclude, then, that the possibility of establishing a national health program depends on the possibility of strengthening the labor movement. Without a stronger labor movement, the likelihood of a national health program is greatly diminished.

Yet the U.S. labor movement is weaker than it has been in its entire history. Does this mean that it is impossible to establish a national health program? Not necessarily. History can change rapidly.

The collapse of the Soviet system took place in less than two years, and a characteristic of all major capitalist countries today is their political instability. The governments of all the advanced capitalist countries are in deep trouble; the popularity of their leaders is at an all-time low. The current situation in the United States confirms this state of affairs.

People want change, profound change. And they see government as unresponsive to their needs. The end of the Cold War opens many new possibilities: this is the end of one era and the beginning of a new one. The greatest challenge we face is to provide information, to assist those who organize, and to help them realize that there is more that unites them than divides them. Which leads me to the topic of the final chapter, the need to eradicate classism, sexism, and racism in our health care institutions and our populations.

5

CLASSISM, RACISM, AND SEXISM IN THE HEALTH SECTOR

THE CLASS, RACE, AND GENDER COMPOSITION OF THE LABOR FORCE IN THE HEALTH SECTOR

When most scientific bibliographies refer to those who work in the health sector, they generally are referring to doctors. Yet doctors make up only a very small percentage of the labor force in this sector. Table 5-1 shows the occupational structure of the health sector labor force, and its class, race, and gender composition.

At the top we find the upper-middle-class, predominantly white male physicians, as well as senior administrators, dentists, pharmacists, and so on. The middle group is lower middle class and predominantly female. African-Americans are represented

Table 5-1

Occupational Structure of the U.S. Labor Force in the Health Sector (by percent)

	Percentage of Health Sector Labor Force		Percentage of Jobs in Category Held by Women		Percentage of Jobs in Category Held by African-Americans	
	1970	1987	1970	1987	1970	1987
Physicians	7.3	6.9	6.9	18.2	3.0	4.0
Dentists, pharmacists	6.5	5.0	7.9	9.2	2.5	3.0
Administrators, scientists	3.5	9.0	30.0	42.0	5.0	6.0
Therapists	3.4	3.0	76.0	80.0	7.0	8.0
Technologists, technicians	8.0	9.0	69.0	72.0	18.0	19.0
Registered nurses	17.1	11.1	97.0	97.0	6.0	9.0
Clerical workers	8.0	14.0	93.0	94.0	19.0	20.0
Nonclerical workers	46.0	44.0	82.0	84.0	22.0	23.0
Total	**100.0**	**100.0**	**72.0**	**78.0**	**18.0**	**22.0**

Table 5-2

Ratio of Earnings of the Average Physician to Those of the Average Wage Earner, 1990

United Kingdom	2.8
Sweden	2.9
West Germany	5.1
France	4.8
Canada	5.2
United States	6.0

---

far beyond their representation in the population as a whole. This group includes registered nurses, therapists, technologists, and technicians, among others. The bottom group is the working class; it includes clerical and service workers and is also predominantly female, with African-Americans even more over-represented than in the middle group.

A key characteristic of this labor force is the enormous difference between the incomes earned by the professionals and the incomes earned by the working class. No other advanced capitalist country exhibits such a disparity. In the United States, for instance, the average net income (i.e., income after taxes) of the chief executives of the large insurance companies is $890,000, while the average medical specialist makes $850,000 (net) and the average generalist $150,000 (net). The average nurse, on the other hand, makes $28,000 and the average cleaning woman in the hospital makes $16,000. The income ratio between the top and bottom is 55 to 1. As Table 5-2 shows, no other advanced capitalist country has the huge income differentials that we see in the United States.

The majority of workers in the health sector are poorly paid. If we compare the standard of living of the labor force in the health sector with that of the labor force as a whole in 1990, we find that the standard of living was much lower for health work-

Figure 5-1
Standard of Living of the U.S. Labor Force and the Health Sector Labor Force (by percent)

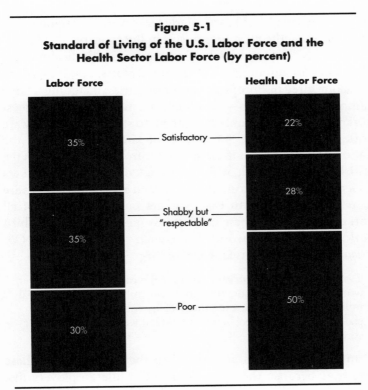

ers: while 30 percent of the overall labor force was considered "poor," 50 percent of the health sector labor force fell into this category (see Figure 5-1). "Poor" is defined here as a family that has just enough income to buy the minimum required food, has no money for recreation, lives in low-quality and low-rent housing, has no savings, drives a used car or uses public transportation, and purchases new clothes only every three years.

Health care workers are both poorly paid and poorly organized, with less than 18 percent belonging to unions. Local 1199 is the largest union among health care workers. Because of the large number of minorities in the health sector labor force, these unions have always been particularly sensitive to civil rights issues and are among the most progressive in the country.

These class, race, and gender characteristics of the health sector labor force are not unique to the United States. Large sectors of this labor force in Europe are also minorities, including a large number of immigrants—what are euphemistically called "guest workers," whose visas only allow them to stay as long as they are working. For example, 43 percent of kitchen workers in the National Health Service in Great Britain are immigrants from the British Commonwealth, while 40 percent of all hospital workers in Germany and 60 percent in Switzerland are immigrants, as are 38 percent of all health care workers (and 24 percent of all workers) in France. These men and women represent the third world within the first world. The French weekly *Le Nouvel Observateur* noted the consequences of this:

> Two million foreign workers [in France] means two million fewer worker votes at election time and two million fewer potential militants in the factories: in other words, a quarter of the working class is "denationalized," and its political weight diminished accordingly.[1]

Immigrant workers are critical to the economies of these countries because they provide labor, while employers like them because they are a "docile" working class. They can be expelled at will, there are always more waiting to take their places, and because they are not citizens, they have no role in political life.

Racism plays a critical role in dividing the working class, a racism that is frequently stimulated by employers' associations and their political instruments. A clear example is Bethlehem Steel. Until the late 1950s, if you visited one of its Baltimore mills, you would see that the foremen were German, the skilled workers were Italian, and the unskilled workers were African-American. Such ethnic and racial divisions were deliberately maintained in order to separate and weaken the working class. The absence of class discourse and an emphasis, instead, on race divides rather than unites the working class. The consequences of this division in both political and scientific institutions are many.

CLASSISM AND RACISM AND THEIR IMPLICATIONS FOR HEALTH POLICY

I had the privilege of being the senior health advisor to the Reverend Jesse Jackson in his Democratic presidential primary campaigns in both 1984 and 1988. As such I could see first-hand how the political establishment of this country responds to issues of class and race.

In 1984, Jackson ran as the minority candidate—the voice of the poor and the excluded. His message was "Our time has come." It was a message of moral outrage, a denunciation and a demand for inclusion. It was primarily the voice of black America, of the minority. The mainstream press responded positively. It saw Jackson as the country's conscience: white America needed to be sensitive to the special plight of the minorities, in particular blacks.

In 1988, however, Jesse Jackson ran as the voice of the working class—not only the black working class, but of Hispanics, Asians, and whites. He emphasized class as well as race, and tried to make white workers aware that they had far more in common with their black fellow workers than with their white bosses—that class could be a *uniting* element. When Jackson was asked how he planned to make white workers aware of their interests, he responded, "By calling on their class interests."

In the area of health policy, Jackson's strategies in 1984 and 1988 were also different. In 1984, the call was for more health programs for the most vulnerable people, particularly minorities. In 1988, however, Jackson called for a universal and comprehensive health program that would respond to the needs of *all* Americans. The issue of universality was at the center of the program.

The response of the establishment was very different in 1988 than it had been in 1984. It quickly realized that Jackson's class appeal might invoke a positive response not only from the 11 percent of the population that was African-American, but from the majority of Americans, the working class. Indeed, Jackson won in the primaries in most cities with populations over 100,000, creating what a *New York Times* editorial called "a political earthquake." Here was a major political figure who used explicitly class discourse that emphasized exploitation and economic violence. The capitalist class felt threatened and summoned all its resources to stop Jackson. Those of us who were close to him even feared for his life.

CLASSISM AND RACISM IN THE HEALTH, SCIENTIFIC, GOVERNMENT, AND ACADEMIC INSTITUTIONS

The absence of "class" is also evident in the scientific and government institutions of the United States. The U.S. government collects statistics about mortality rates and causes of death by race, gender, and region, but not by class. This is not the case in the majority of developed capitalist countries. In fact, most Western European governments, with the active encouragement of the European office of the World Health Organization (WHO), have made the reduction of the differentials in mortality rates by class a primary objective. In the United States, in contrast, there is a deafening silence regarding class mortality differentials. Instead of class, the U.S. government uses race, and lists the reduction of mortality differentials by race as one of its top five objectives.

Why does the United States use race rather than class in its mortality statistics, and why is class a nonexistent category in all of our other health statistics? The answers to these questions are critical to understanding the connection between science, ideology, and politics in this country.

But first I must emphasize that the government's objective of reducing race mortality differentials is of course very important. African-Americans have higher mortality rates and shorter life expectancies than white Americans. In 1988, for instance, life expectancy at birth was 75.5 years for whites, but only 69.5 years for blacks. On average, blacks live 2,160 fewer days than whites. Blacks also generally have higher mortality rates than whites, and for many causes of death the mortality differential between blacks and whites is increasing. Alarming reports of these trends have appeared in the press and in medical publications. But although we should certainly support the government's objective of reducing these differentials, the fact is that the government will not be able to do this if it focuses only on race. In fact, even without these race differentials, most blacks would still have higher mortality rates than the median or mean rate of the population as a whole. In order to understand this, we must rediscover the silenced category of class.

There are classes in the United States, and how people live and die depends largely on the class they belong to. On one of the few occasions (in 1986) that the government did collect information on mortality rates for one of the most important causes of mortality—heart disease—by class, the results showed a strong correlation between mortality and class. People who belong to the working class (in this case defined as the census categories of operators and service workers) were more likely to die of heart disease than people belonging to the managerial and professional classes. Figure 5-2 shows mortality rates by occupation.

In the 1986 data, the mortality rate for heart disease was 2.3 times higher for blue-collar workers than for managers and professionals. This class differential is much greater than the white/black mortality differential: the heart disease mortality rate was 1.2 times greater for black males than for white males and 1.5 times greater for black females than for white females. And the class mortality differentials between, say, blue-collar or service workers and corporate lawyers increased during the 1980s—even more than did race differentials.[2]

The key point here is that the growing class mortality differentials, which are ignored by the government and the media, are

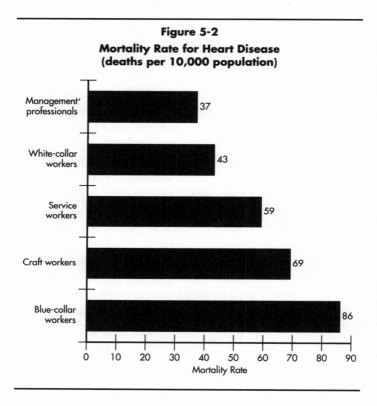

Figure 5-2
Mortality Rate for Heart Disease
(deaths per 10,000 population)

primarily responsible for the growing race mortality differentials, not the other way around. This is because the overwhelming majority of blacks (and other minorities) belong to the low-paid sectors of the working class. As we saw in Chapter 2, in the 1980s there was a growing class polarization, with a reduction in the size of the middle (well-paid) sectors of the working population and a rapid growth in the low-paid, unskilled sectors of the working class. The working class came to be increasingly made up of nonunionized, poorly paid, and part-time workers, with a preponderance of minorities and women. These low-wage earners are a heterogeneous group—blacks, Hispanics, whites, men, women—whose standards of living are rapidly deteriorating. By 1984, 40 percent of the population received only 15.7 percent of the total income, the lowest figure since data collection began in 1974. In contrast, the wealthiest 20 percent received 42.9 percent of the total income, the highest ever. It is this growing disparity of wealth and income that explains the race differentials in mortality.

The evidence is overwhelming that class is an extremely important category for understanding the lives and deaths of the U.S. population. Why, then, do the government and the media focus on race and ignore class? Why is the United States the only major developed capitalist country that does not collect mortality statistics by class? In order to answer these questions, we have to return to our earlier discussion: not only does the United States have classes, but the capitalist class is extremely powerful and the working class very weak. The absence of class analysis and class discourse is a victory for the capitalist class, which encourages the myth of the "middle-class society." The capitalist class emphasizes race rather than class as a means to keep white workers on its side. For instance, mortality statistics that show that whites have better health indicators than blacks suggest that white workers are more similar to their white bosses than they are to black workers. Because of racism, blacks have higher mortality indicators than whites within each class and within each occupational category. That is why it is important to publish mortality statistics by race, standardized by class. But the publication of mortality statistics by race alone is not only unscientific, it is an ideological statement. It assumes—as the federal government does—that race is the most important category by which to divide our population. This assumption is of course wrong: it divides rather than unites people who, in fact, have far more that unites than divides them. Workers, white or black, have more similarities than differences in their ways of living and dying.

This perception of our reality became clear to me during the Democratic presidential primaries in 1988. As I noted above, the political and media establishments kept defining Jackson as the "black candidate" in order to isolate him and limit his appeal to a small constituency—the black minority—which, being the most exploited, is the most progressive sector of our population. The establishment was afraid of Jackson's class appeal. It did not want to recognize him as the voice of *all* the disenfranchised, white and black. As Dan Rather and Walter Cronkite reported during the Democratic convention, where 30 percent of the delegates were backing Jackson, "The fact that he [Jackson] is so powerful frightens some people. I would count ourselves among those individuals. We watched the rise of people who seemed to be speaking for the underprivileged for a long time and then when they got power things went awry."[3] But Jackson's power did not come from his personality alone; it came from his class message, and it did indeed threaten class privileges. The U.S. establishment has always repressed the class positions of the dominated classes.

Class repression takes place in all spheres of life, including our academic and scientific institutions, and effective repression silences any form of class analysis or discourse. Let me share an example. I recently prepared an analysis of morbidity and mortality differentials in the United States by class and race, and criticized the government for not collecting or publishing mortality statistics by class. I submitted this article to two major U.S. medical journals, the *New England Journal of Medicine* and the *Journal of the American Medical Association (JAMA)*. Both rejected the article with arguments that they considered scientific but I considered highly ideological. For example, the *JAMA* reviewer indicated that while I had shown that the working class had more sickness and higher mortality rates than other classes, I had not *disproved* the possibility that people were in the working class because they were sicker to begin with. In other words, the reviewer suggested that rather than social conditions explaining disease, biological conditions determined social conditions. And he imposed *his* views by repressing *my* views (rejecting my article). *JAMA* has published special issues on blacks, Hispanics, and women, but it is unlikely that it will publish a special issue on class. Yet when I submitted my article to the *Lancet,* the most prestigious medical journal in Europe, it published it right away, giving it great prominence and including the supportive editorial entitled "The U.S.: Not a Classless Society." An effective way of repressing views is by suppressing their publication in scientific journals. This greatly damages the nature of the scientific project. Our knowledge about the causes of mortality is seriously hindered by the suppression of information that could shed light on the probabilities of living and dying in this country.

CLASS, RACE, AND GENDER POWER IN THE HEALTH TEAM

At the beginning of this chapter I noted that most physicians are white, upper-middle-class males, that most nurses are white, lower-middle-class females, and that most workers in the health sector are female and often minority. This class, race, and gender hierarchy in the health team reproduces the pattern of relations in a Victorian family. Florence Nightingale, the founder of nursing, referred to the duties of the nurse as being like the wife of the doctor, the mother of the patient, and the master of the health aides. We see, then, the physician as the center of the health team, with the nurse as his appendix. The consequences of this hierarchical relationship are many. One is the dominance of *curing* over *caring.* Physicians are trained in curing, with an emphasis on technological intervention. Nurses, on the other hand, are trained in caring—in taking care of patients. Because relationships in the health sector reproduce the dominant class and gender relations in the larger society, curing by white upper-middle-class males becomes more prestigious than caring, the function carried out by lower-middle-class females.

Approximately 65 percent of medical expenditures go toward curing, even though most diseases are chronic, for which the appropriate intervention is caring. The nurse, therefore, could be the coordinator of the health team. But the possibility of this is

nil, not because there is no rationale for such a change in responsibility, but because it would go against the class and gender
power relations in our society.

Let me finish this chapter by referring again to the relationship
among class, race, and science. The corporate class is the most
class-conscious of all classes. It does not tolerate class threats. It
does tolerate, encourage, and coopt race and gender practices.
Therefore women and members of minority groups have been
sought by the establishment to legitimize its commitment to
diversity. To be politically correct today means to have women
and minorities at the center of political and academic life. The
gender and race composition of the corporate class and its allied
forces has also become more inclusive.

But, as I have shown in this book, there has been no such
diversity in class terms. The working class remains absent from
political and academic life. Equally important, anti-corporate
and radical views that question the nature of class relations are
systematically excluded from our major value-generating systems—be they the media, academia, or political institutions.
Those of you who are African-American, Hispanic, or members
of other minorities will be sought after, and all types of positions
will be given to you—top government and academic positions,
directorships of boards—if you are willing to conform to the class
relations of this country. If, however, you rebel against these class
relations, you will be discriminated against. But you will be doing
far more for those whom you want to serve—the majority of your
people—than if you adapt yourself to our class-dominated institutions.

Finally, to all of you—whites, African-Americans, Hispanics,
and the many other groups and minorities that make up the
beautiful rainbow that is the United States: if you want to serve
our people, to protect their health and cure their diseases, you
must learn from them as well, learn from the enormous wisdom
that they have acquired through their daily lives. You must also
share with them the information that you, in your life, have been

able to obtain from documents, books, and printed materials. Assist them in the process of organizing, help them recover their political, social, academic, and health care institutions, so that the government of these institutions becomes, as President Abraham Lincoln put it so beautifully, "of the people, by the people, for the people."

NOTES

INTRODUCTION

1. Vincent Canby, "A Blue-Collar Comedy in English, Subtitled," *New York Times*, 12 February 1993.
2. For a discussion of the importance of health care issues in the 1992 presidential election campaign, see Vicente Navarro, *The Politics of the U.S. Welfare State: The Case of Medicine* (New York: Basil Blackwell, forthcoming in 1994).

CHAPTER 1: WHY THE U.S. HEALTH CARE SYSTEM DOES NOT RESPOND TO PEOPLE'S NEEDS

1. Quoted in Benjamin DeMott, *The Imperial Middle: Why Americans Can't Think Straight About Class* (New York: William Morrow, 1990), p. 9.
2. As confirmed by the class self-identification survey conducted by the National Opinion Research Center, published in *Public Opinion: Social Class*, for 1980, 1984, 1986, 1990, and 1992. See also Vicente Navarro, "The Middle Class—A Useful Myth," *The Nation*, 23 March 1992, p. 1.
3. Paul Samuelson, *Economics* (8th ed.; New York: McGraw-Hill, 1972), p. 110.

4. U.S. Senate, Committee on Government Operations, *Disclosure of Corporate Ownership* (Washington, DC: Government Printing Office, 1973).
5. As reported by M. Mintz, "Eight Institutions Control Most of the Top Firms," *Washington Post,* 6 January 1974, pp. A1 and A6.
6. Karl Marx and Friedrich Engels, *The Communist Manifesto* (New York: Monthly Review Press, 1964), p. 6.
7. Vicki Kemper and Viveca Novak, "What's Blocking Health Care Reform?" *Common Cause Magazine* 18, no. 1 (January/February/March 1992): 8-13, 25.
8. Vicente Navarro, *The Politics of the Welfare State.*
9. "Health Plan Progress," *New York Times,* 7 April 1974, p. E16.
10. Kemper and Novak, "What's Blocking Health Care Reform?"
11. Abraham Flexner, *Universities: American, English, German* (rev. ed., New York: Oxford University Press, 1930), p. 180.
12. R.M. MacIver, *Academic Freedom in Our Time* (New York: Goodwin Press, 1967), p. 78.
13. J.K. Galbraith, *The New Industrial State* (Boston: Houghton Mifflin, 1967), p. 370.
14. N. M. Pusey, *Age of the Scholars: Observations on Education in a Troubled Decade* (Cambridge, MA: Harvard University Press, 1963), p. 171.
15. Ralph Miliband, *The State in Capitalist Society: An Analysis of the Western System of Power* (London: Weidenfeld and Nicolson, 1969), p. 20.
16. William H. Hartley and William S. Vincent, *American Civics* (Orlando, FL: Harcourt Brace Jovanovich, 1987), p. 434.
17. *New York Times,* 24 September 1992.
18. U.S. Congress, Office of the Budget, *Economic Implications of Rising Health Care Costs,* October 1992, p. 37.
19. E. E. Schattschneider, *The Sovereign People: A Realistic View of Democracy in America* (New York: Holt, Rinehart, & Winston, 1960), p. 31.
20. New York Times/CBS Poll, August 1991.
21. Senator Jay Rockefeller, speech to the Conference of the Health Alliance of America, Summer 1991.

CHAPTER 2: CLASS STRUGGLE IN THE HEALTH SECTOR DURING THE REAGAN/BUSH YEARS

1. Reported in *El Pais,* 14 August 1983.
2. Gallup Poll Reports, September 1984.
3. Edward Snyder, Testimony to the House Budget Committee of the U.S. Congress, August 1978.
4. *New York Times,* 24 October 1978.

5. *Economic Report of the Council of Economic Advisors to the President of the United States* (Washington, DC: 1986), p. 14.
6. Senator Daniel Patrick Moynihan, Declarations in the Budget Committee, January 1981.
7. U.S. Congress, Senate, *The Environmental Conditions of the United States* (Washington, DC: Government Printing Office, 1982).
8. Military expenditures are much larger than Defense Department expenditures. They include Veterans Administration and NASA expenditures, a large part of the Department of Energy expenditures and foreign aid, and a large percentage of the national debt.

CHAPTER 3: THE DEMOCRATIC PARTY AND THE FUTURE OF HEALTH CARE IN THE UNITED STATES

1. Harris Poll, 5 January 1993.
2. Paul Ellwood, *Medical Care* 9 (1971): 291.
3. Alain Enthoven and Richard Kronick, *New England Journal of Medicine* 320 (1989): 94.
4. "Health Care Reform: Not Journalistically Viable," *Extra* 6, no. 5 (July-August 1993).
5. Cited in Theodore R. Marmor, "Commentary on Canadian Health Insurance: Lessons for the United States," *International Journal of Health Services* 23, no. 1 (1993): 45-62.

CHAPTER 4: CLASS POWER AND HEALTH CARE: WHY THE UNITED STATES IS DIFFERENT

1. Gosta Esping-Andersen, "Power and Distributional Regimes," *Politics and Society* 14, no. 2 (1985): 223-56.
2. Ibid., p. 229.
3. G. Esping-Andersen and W. Korpi, "Social Policy as Class Politics in Post-War Capitalism: Scandinavia, Austria, and Germany" in *Order and Conflict in Contemporary Capitalism,* ed. J.H. Gadthorpe (New York: Oxford University Press, 1984), Table B2, p. 198.
4. Ibid., p. 231.
5. Ibid. and W. Korpi, *The Democratic Class Struggle* (Boston: Routledge and Kegan Paul, 1983).
6. G. Esping-Andersen, *Politics Against Markets: The Social Democratic Road to Power* (Princeton, NJ: Princeton University Press, 1985).
7. Mike Davis, *Prisoners of the American Dream* (London: Verso, 1986).
8. G. Therborn, "When, How, and Why Does a State Become a Welfare State?"

Paper presented at the ECPR Workshop on Comparative Study of Distribution and Social Policy in Advanced Industrialized Nations, Freiburg, 20-25 March 1983.

9. J.A. Meyer and M.E. Levin, "Poverty and Social Welfare: An Agenda for Change," *Inquiry* 23, no. 2 (1986): 122-33.

10. W. Green, "A National Health Program for a Stronger America," *American Federalist* 59, no. 6 (1952).

11. C. Renner and V. Navarro, "Why Is Our Population of Uninsured and Underinsured Persons Growing?" *International Journal of Health Services* 19 (1989): 433-42.

12. M. G. Taylor, *Health Insurance and Canadian Public Policy* (Montreal: McGill University Press, 1978).

13. Organization for Economic Cooperation and Development, *Measuring Health Care 1960-1983. Expenditures, Costs and Performance*, OECD Social Policy Studies No. 2 (1985).

14. "A Left Majority in the EEC," *New Socialist* 33, no. 4 (1985).

15. This refers to the top twenty-three members of the Organization of Economic Cooperation and Development (OECD). See G. Therborn, "The Prospects of Labour and the Transformation of Advanced Capitalism," *New Left Review* 145 (1984).

16. Newsnight poll, February 10; *Guardian,* 11 February 1986; cited in *Marxism Today,* March 1986. See also Vicente Navarro, "Where Is the Popular Mandate?" *New England Journal of Medicine* 307 (1982): 1516-18.

17. Leo Panitch, *Working Class Politics in Crisis* (London: Verso, 1986), p. 7.

18. Quoted in Ellen Meiksins Wood, *The Retreat from Class* (London: Verso, 1986), p. 182.

19. Quoted in M. Pertschuck, *Revolt Against Regulation* (Berkeley, CA: University of California Press, 1982), p. 57.

20. P. Anderson, "European Social Democracy," *Against the Current* 1, no. 6 (1986) 21-28.

CHAPTER 5: CLASSISM, RACISM, AND SEXISM IN THE HEALTH SECTOR

1. M. Busquet, *Le Nouvel Observateur,* 23 August 1982.

2. Vicente Navarro, "Race or Class Versus Race and Class: Mortality Differentials in the United States," *The Lancet,* 17 November 1990, p. 1238.

3. CBS report of the Democratic Party Convention, 1988.

SOURCES FOR FIGURES AND TABLES

Figure 1-1: From David Himmelstein and Steffie Woolhandler, *The National Health Program Chartbook* (Cambridge, MA: The Center for National Health Program Studies, Harvard Medical School, 1992).

Figure 1-2: From Himmelstein and Woolhandler, *The National Health Program Chartbook.*

Figure 1-3: Calculated from U.S. Bureau of the Census, *1990 Census of the Population.*

Figure 1-4: Calculated from individual national and World Bank reports, 1989, 1990, 1991, and 1992.

Figure 1-5: From Teresa Amott, *Caught in the Crisis: Women and the U.S. Economy Today* (New York: Monthly Review Press, 1993); data from Robert S. McIntyre, *Inequality and the Federal Budget Deficit* (Washington, DC: Citizens for Tax Justice, 1991), p. 7.

Figure 1-6: Vicente Navarro, "Analysis of the Social Class and Gender Composition of the Board of Trustees in the Health Sector in the United States," paper presented to the Xth Annual Congress of the International Association of Health Policy, Bologna, Italy, 1992. In this study I have included the category clerical and sales workers under lower middle class rather than working class (as in Figure 1-3), because of the statistical requirements of the study.

Figure 1-7: Adapted and updated from Grace Ziem, "Evolution of the Class, Race, and Gender Composition of the Medical Student Body in the United States," Ph.D. diss., Harvard University School of Public Health, 1982.

Figure 1-8: Navarro, "Analysis of the Social Class and Gender Composition of the Board of Trustees in the Health Sector in the United States." Because of the statistical requirements of this study, clerical and office workers in the working class (see Figure 1-3) were instead included in the lower middle class.

Figure 2-1: From Amott, *Caught in the Crisis,* p. 120; data from McIntyre, *Inequality and the Federal Budget Deficit,* p. 12. Figures are spending changes as a percent of GNP times the FY 1990 GNP.

Figure 2-2: Himmelstein and Woolhandler, *The National Health Program Chartbook.*

Figure 2-3: From G.J. Schieber, "Health Expenditures in Major Industrialized Countries, 1960-1987," *Health Care Financing Review* 11, no. 4 (1990): 159-67.

Figure 3-1: OECD 1990.

Figure 3-2: OECD 1990.

Figure 3-3: Vicente Navarro, David Himmelstein, and Steffie Woolhandler, *The Jackson National Health Program* (The National Rainbow Coalition, 1988).

Figure 3-4: Congressional Research Service, *Costs and Effects of Extending Health Insurance Coverage* (Washington, DC: Education and Labor Serial No.

100-EE, 1988): 46; cited in Robert J. Blendon and Tracey Stelzer Hyams, *Reforming the System* (New York: Faulkner Gray, 1992).

Figure 5-1: AFL-CIO Research Institute, 1990.

Figure 5-2: Vicente Navarro, "Class or Race or Class and Race: Mortality Differentials in the United States," *Lancet,* 17 November 1990.

Table 1-2: From Himmelstein and Woolhandler, *The National Health Program Chartbook.*

Table 1-3: *New York Times,* 11 June 1993, p. A22; data from the Center for Responsive Politics and the Federal Election Commission.

Table 1-4: Estimated from U.S. Census, *Current Population Reports. Voting and Registration in the Elections of 1984 and 1988* (Washington, DC: 1990).

Table 2-1: H.E. Freeman et al., "Americans Report on Their Access to Health Care," *Health Forum,* Spring 1987, pp. 6-18.

Table 2-2: Himmelstein and Woolhandler, *The National Health Program Chartbook.*

Table 2-3: Estimated from U.S. Census, *Voting and Registration in the Elections of 1976, 1980, 1984, and 1988,* and from press accounts of popular participation in 1992.

Table 2-4: Vicente Navarro, "The Determinants of Occupational Health Policy. A Case Study: Sweden," *Journal of Health Politics, Policy, and Law* 9, no. 1 (1984): 137-66.

Table 2-5: *The States of the Environment in OECD Member Countries, 1979* (Paris: OECD, 1980).

Table 3-1: Kaiser/Harris Health Insurance Survey, Louis Harris and Associates, April 1992.

Table 4-1: Adapted from G. Esping-Andersen and W. Korpi, "Social Policy as Class Politics in Post-War Capitalism: Scandinavia, Austria, and Germany" in *Order and Conflict in Contemporary Capitalism,* ed. J.H. Gadthorpe (New York: Oxford University Press, 1984), Table B2, p. 198. In all these countries, socialist parties increased their political following and were in power for the whole or parts of this period.

Table 4-2: G. Therborn, "When, How, and Why Does a State Become a Welfare State?" Paper presented at the ECPR Workshop on Comparative Study of Distribution and Social Policy in Advanced Industrialized Nations, Freiburg, 20-25 March 1983.

Table 4-3: OECD, *Measuring Health Care, 1960-1983. Expenditures, Costs, and Performance,* OECD Social Policy Studies No. 2 (1985), Table 2, p. 12.

Table 5-1: Estimated from U.S. Bureau of Labor Statistics reports, various years.

Table 5-2: Organization for Economic Cooperation and Development statistics (Paris: OECD, 1992).

INDEX